AF882661

SOTHIS PRESS

Sothis Press aims to completely reimagine the public domain book with an emphasis on universal access to captivatingly designed print editions. We believe that technology will enable every single book ever published to be perpetually accessible in beautiful print form. Sothis is beauty in ubiquity.

www.sothis.press

1 Waterhouse Square, London, EC1N 2ST

Some Observations on the Contamination of Water by the Poison of Lead and Its Effects on the Human Body

Together With Remarks on Some Other Modes in Which Lead May Be Injurious in Domestic Life

James Bower Harrison

SOTHIS PRESS

ISBN 978-1-0365-0974-3

Some Observations on the Contamination of Water by the Poison of Lead and Its Effects on the Human Body is in the public domain.

This edition is published by Sothis Press © 2023. The company is registered in England and Wales. The Company Number is 14900389.

CONTAMINATION OF WATER

BY THE

POISON OF LEAD.

"Bonum est, fugienda aspicere alieno in malo."—*Publ. Syr.*

It is a good thing to learn caution by the misfortunes of others.

SOME OBSERVATIONS

ON THE

CONTAMINATION OF WATER

BY THE

POISON OF LEAD:

AND

ITS EFFECTS ON THE HUMAN BODY;

TOGETHER WITH

REMARKS ON SOME OTHER MODES IN WHICH LEAD MAY
BE INJURIOUS IN DOMESTIC LIFE.

BY

JAMES BOWER HARRISON,
M.R.C S L., &c. &c.
FORMERLY SURGEON TO THE ARDWICK AND ANCOATS DISPENSARY;
CORRESPONDING MEMBER OF THE EPIDEMIOLOGICAL SOCIETY

LONDON:
JOHN CHURCHILL, PRINCES STREET, SOHO.
MDCCCLII.

BOSTON MEDICAL
LIBRARY

PREFACE.

WHATEVER may be the motives attributed to me by others, I can honestly state that I write what follows for the public good. If I had been anxious to extend my practice as a medical man, I should have chosen any other subject in preference to that upon which I have written. On the other hand, I do not greatly value popular fame, when I find so large a share of patronage bestowed upon those whom I conscientiously believe to be either mistaken in their views, or dishonest in their practice; and I can state, from my own observation, that more applause is commonly received by those, who pander to the prejudices of their patients, than by those who treat them with sincerity and skill.

I do not arrogate to myself any superiority of discrimination or originality of discovery:—I wish only to press on the attention of mankind truths which have been long known, and as long neglected. I anticipate, in fact, no other advantage from this publication than that of contributing something to the good of mankind.

It may appear to some, that I am making protestations of candour which are somewhat unnecessary; but let it be remembered, that whilst the present age is one of great advancement, it is one, also, in which Empiricism has gained an unusual amount of public approbation.

When I commenced preparing these sheets

for the press, I was not aware that Dr. Alderson was about to make the effects of lead the subject of the Lumleian Lectures; nor did I know that a review of the work of Tanquerel Desplanches would appear in the 'Edinburgh Journal of Medicine.' I am glad, however, to welcome these contributions to our knowlege of the subject, and I do not think they have altogether rendered what I have written unnecessary.

HIGHER BROUGHTON;
October, 1852.

CONTAMINATION OF WATER

BY THE

POISON OF LEAD.

The poisonous effects of Lead have been so long known, and been so ably described by a multitude of writers, that it may seem extraordinary at the present day that any one should have the hardihood to publish an account of them. Long ago the pen of Sir George Baker illustrated the subjcet with all the elegance, erudition, and sagacity for which he was so eminently distinguished. Dr. Warren, about the same period, described the colic of lead with a faithfulness of portraiture which left little to be desired. On the Continent, Mérat Andral, and especially Tanquerel Desplanches, have pursued the inquiry with a zeal and ability peculiar, and highly creditable to the diligence and accuracy of the French. To enter now upon a field thus occupied, may require some apology,—it would, indeed, require a very serious apology, if I had any pretensions to follow in their footsteps, and measure the value of their large results by my own humble experience.—I have no such pretensions; but I *do* feel that there is one branch of this subject which has yet to be fully revealed. I know that the profession and the public have yet to be awakened to the insidious poison which lurks in their houses, and is the secret cause of slow disease, issuing in palsy and epilepsy, and in icteric wasting of the body. I know that the contamination of water with lead has been observed even in ancient times; but I am aware that it is only at the present period that the subject has been rightly comprehended, and the danger properly understood. What apology, then, is necessary for an effort to rouse attention, and extend information so desirable to be known!

When I first entered upon the inquiry into the effects of contaminated water, I supposed that it was one of comparatively limited application. I believed that the cases in which people suffered from this cause were few and accidental, and always, in the end, sufficiently apparent to the medical attendant. I now feel convinced that the cases are very numerous, at least in my own neighbourhood, and no doubt also in others. I feel sure that they are often, for a long time, misunderstood and improperly treated, and that deaths arise not unfrequently without the true cause being ever imagined. I know that many persons leave their dwellings under wrong impressions as to the salubrity of their localities, without ever conjecturing that bad water is the real source of their disorders. I am almost afraid of enumerating the cases which have fallen under my own observation, lest, in the relation of the truth, I lay myself open to the appearance of exaggeration. Sterne says, "I would not shake my credit by telling an improbable truth, however indisputable in itself;"[1] and it is certain that it sometimes requires courage to make just statements which may appear in an unfavorable light, and bear a wrong interpretation. I may, however, here say, once for all, that I have rejected all cases which might be open to doubt, or have given them with a proper caution and admission of their uncertainty.—No advantage could arise from making assertions which would be eventually discovered incorrect,

[1] Tristram Shandy.

and which could never advance the cause they were brought forward to support.

Owing to the cheapness of lead, and owing to its softness and the easy manner in which it may be rolled into sheets, it is largely used in the arts in the formation of cisterns and pipes; nor is its value less in the combinations into which it enters, and on which it bestows properties of singular beauty and utility. It is necessary, however, to bear in mind that lead may exercise poisonous influences on the body, and that a constant and even suspicious regard should be always directed to the possibility of danger from its employment.

So numerous, indeed, are the uses of lead, and consequently so many the channels through which it may be undesignedly taken, that it would be almost tedious to enumerate them,—still more, to point out at length all the circumstances, even of importance and interest, which are connected with the inquiry. There is one part of this subject, however, which, as I have stated, is so important in itself, that I have thought it necessary to call particular attention to it, for, though it has been very long known, it has been perpetually lost sight of, or neglected. A very great while ago it was discovered that water, which had stood in contact with lead, sometimes became poisonous; but as this result was not universally noticed, and the precise circumstances on which it depended were not clearly ascertained, it never became so fully known, nor attracted so much attention, as, in reality, it deserved, and, indeed, required.—The history of the progress of knowledge on this subject is so replete with interest, and so necessary for the right understanding of what follows, that I may be excused for very briefly entering upon it.

Every one must have noticed the white crust which forms on the sides of leaden cisterns in which water is contained. This could not escape attention even in ancient times, nor was it long before its poisonous nature was ascertained.

Vitruvius, the Roman architect, who is supposed to have been contemporary with Cæsar and Augustus, forbids the use of this metal for conducting water, because *ceruse*, (carbonate of lead,) he says, is formed on it, which is hurtful to the human body.[1]

Galen also noticed the prejudicial effects of lead in imparting muddiness to water. These statements were repeated by succeeding observers; but it was not until Dr. Lambe of Warwick entered upon the inquiry in 1803, that a more minute investigation of the subject was made. Dr. Lambe came

[1] De Architectura, lib. viii, c. vii. The passage alluded to is as follows: "Multo salubrior ex tubulis aqua, quam per fistulas: quod per plumbum videtur esse ideo vitiosa, quod ex eo cerussa nascitur: hæc autem dicitur esse nocens corporibus humanis. Ita si quod ex eo procreatur id est vitiosum non est dubium quin ipsum quoque non sit salubre."

to the conclusion that most spring waters were capable of corroding and dissolving lead, and therefore that they could not with impunity be kept in such receptacles. Spring water is known to contain various saline ingredients, and it was natural enough to suppose that the solvent power of the water was produced by their presence.

Guyton-Morveau next entered upon the inquiry, and pursued the investigation in a more correct and scientific manner. Curiously enough he arrived at conclusions directly opposite to those of Dr. Lambe. He found, from his own researches, that distilled water, which is the purest of waters, acted most rapidly on lead, and he concluded that the corrosive influence of the water was in direct proportion to its purity. The saline matter contained in spring water he considered a means of preventing its action upon lead.

A few years afterwards, Dr. Thomson of

Glasgow again maintained that spring waters were capable of corroding lead, but he thought that the lead was not dissolved by the water, and could be easily separated by filtration. In this state of the question Dr. Christison of Edinburgh entered upon the inquiry.

Dr. Christison is known to be a most able and accurate chemist, and his researches must be esteemed particularly valuable in relation to all questions of a toxicological nature.

Dr. Christison found that pure distilled, or rain water, if not deprived of its gases, and not excluded from the air, has a rapid action upon lead, and, on the other hand, that hard spring waters have little or no influence. He was induced to suppose that the protection which the lead derived was from the saline ingredients in the water, and arose from their forming insoluble compounds with the lead.

The salts which prevent the action of water on lead he considered to be those which form insoluble salts of lead, as the muriates, the sulphates, and the phosphates.[1] Now it will easily be understood that old lead, the surface of which has been gradually acted upon in this manner, will be less susceptible of the influence of water than recent lead. Hence he found that old cisterns or pipes are less capable of contaminating water than those which are new.

Lately an attempt has been made, principally by writers connected with the Board of Health, to controvert the statements of Dr. Christison, and revive the notion that

[1] It appears that the preserving power of the neutral salts depends on their acids forming insoluble salts with lead. Thus the protecting powers of the acetate of soda, nitrate of potass, muriate of soda, sulphate of lime, arseniate of soda, and phosphate of soda, &c., are inversely, as the solubility of the acetate, nitrate, muriate, sulphate, arseniate, and phosphate of lead. (See Christison on Poisons, 1845, p. 521.)

spring water is the most effective in its action on lead, It seems odd that a point which may be determined by experiment, should form a matter of controversy at the present time. I think, however, there can be little doubt but that the views maintained by Dr. Christison are essentially correct. At the same time it is desirable, as Dr. Christison's experiments were chiefly made on the waters in the neighbourhood of Edinburgh, that the spring waters which exist in other parts should be submitted to careful investigation.[1] I am informed by Dr. Christison, that, when leisure is afforded,

[1] In a letter which Dr. Christison did me the favour to send me, he says, after alluding to his published writings: "I have done nothing since to extend my inquiries further than that I have taken every opportunity of examining the water in any remarkable cases which have come in my way, either as to its action or non-action on lead. All these cases I have found to range themselves according to the principles previously adopted by me from experiment, with one exception. And that is the case of spring water containing very little else than muriates. This is a very un-

he will pursue the inquiry into greater detail.

These remarks may possibly have been a little tedious to those not interested in the history of the chemical part of the question; but they serve to show, in the best manner, the true position of the subject. I must repeat, then, that soft water, or otherwise pure distilled or rain water, not deprived of its gases, nor excluded from the air, acts rapidly on lead, especially when the lead is recent. On the other hand, when the water contains many salts, as hard spring-water,—particularly when these are such as the sulphates or phosphates,—there is little or no effect produced. When the lead is old and already coated by the action of the salts,

common sort of water in Scotland. I have only met with one spring of the kind. It would appear from that instance that it is very difficult to render the water inactive in relation to lead; and that, unlike what happens with other waters, some lead is permanently *dissolved*, probably in the form of chloride."

the effect is still less. Some spring waters, however, are sufficiently pure to affect lead, and others may do so by virtue of the peculiarity of their constituent salts.

Here, then, at length we see the reason of the discrepancy of opinion, and of the slowness with which the truth became known. Owing to the difference which exists in the hardness of water, different results attended the experience of those who made use of lead as a receptacle for water; and a want of nicety and accuracy of inquiry prevented a fair revelation of the circumstances upon which the contamination depended.

Thus some found that they could tàke with impunity water which had stood in leaden vessels, and others, who had a softer kind of water contained in similar receptaeles, suffered the most formidable diseases. Nothing, then, can be more interesting and important than the progress of knowledge on this subject, for it shows us how gradually the true position of a fact known at the time of Cæsar and Augustus was brought to light, and the difficulties which obscured it laid aside.

Even the talented and erudite Sir George Baker, notwithstanding the ingenuity and ability with which he pursued his investigations into the effects of lead, does not seem to have had very clear notions as to the action of lead on water. His experiments, indeed, did not bring him to any certain conclusions. He kept some Thames water and spring water in leaden pipes, and agitated the contents almost daily for two months, but he was not able to discover any lead in it. He also examined other specimens; amongst the rest water which had been kept a fortnight "in an old rusty leaden pipe, long used for the purpose of conveying water."[1] Some water, also collected from the hollows of a leaden covering of a church,

[1] Med.-Chir. Trans., vol. i, p. 292.

which he examined, showed no indications of lead; "the caution, therefore," he continues, "of Vitruvius and of Galen, *as likewise that of Aëtius (who condemns the use of rain water which has flowed down from a roof covered with lead)* could not but appear to me unnecessary except in a case where a quantity of vegetable acid might be supposed to render the metal dissoluble in water." He, however, admits, a little further on, that Dr. Heberden had shown him some water which had been kept twelve years on bits of lead, and in which there was a copious white precipitate both at the bottom and on the sides of the vessel, and that this precipitate he discovered to be lead.

It is evident that these inquiries were not made with that accuracy of detail which distinguishes the researches of modern chemists, and consequently doubt and uncertainty prevailed respecting questions of great practical value.

In investigations relating to the contamination of water, it is desirable that a medical man should himself visit the pump or well from which the water is usually taken. He can thus readily satisfy himself whether the former be of lead. Pumps with leaden spouts are generally made of lead, although they may be neatly boxed round with wood. If painted, the spout may be cut with a strong knife, and the bright metallic surface will easily be seen. The pumps which are contained in the interior of houses, and which raise water to different parts of the house, are generally of lead, and the pipes which connect them are of the same material.

In the larger houses in my own neighbourhood, especially in the new ones, the pumps are of this kind, and the water which they convey is generally contaminated; but as these pumps convey spring water, and not soft water, the contamination is less than it otherwise might be. To examine it, as

I have stated, the first water drawn in the morning should be made the subject of experiment. The pumps which are placed *out of doors* may either be of lead or not, but even those which are of wood and iron (the tree, as it is called, being bored,) may have lead pipes in connection with them. If we have reason, therefore, to suspect that lead may exist in the water, we should test it, whether or not the pump be of lead. A very frequent source of mischief is, however, the drinking of soft water from a leaden cistern. This water is generally brought so conveniently into the kitchen or scullery, that there is always a strong temptation for domestics to make use of it for culinary purposes, particularly to fill the kettle at breakfast or at tea-time. People generally imagine, and almost always tell me, that they could easily distinguish the soft from the hard water, but I question their capability of doing so under all circumstances; and I have certainly known those mistaken who have pretended to the most discrimination.

It is not easy to obtain an admission from domestics when they are in the habit of using soft water, so that the truth, in many cases, is not readily discovered. When they are questioned upon this subject in a manner which implies that they have done wrong, I fear the wish to escape blame has a share in preventing the real case being made known. It is well understood that soft water is better adapted than hard water for the purpose of making infusions, so that, besides the convenience attending the employment of the former, it is often preferred from this particular quality. But I would wish to dwell especially on the temptation which often exists to use soft water for the sake of convenience, for I am sure that this is a very important consideration. Now, modern luxury has introduced a dangerous contrivance, which has tended still further to induce the ignorant domestic to substitute the soft water for that of the spring. In many houses boilers are placed behind the kitchen fire-places, which are supplied from the leaden cisterns with soft water, in such a manner that a tap by the side of the fire-place affords a ready and constant supply of hot water. How much more easy, then, to fill the kettle with this water when the servants rise late in the morning, than to obtain water from the spring; and how much quicker is water made to boil which is already hot, than when taken cold and fresh from a well or a pump! I have conversed with many servants on this point, and they have mostly confessed to having used it, unconscious of its deleterious nature, and imagining that blackness was the only possible objection. Two of the worst cases of lead colic, I have ever met with, have arisen from the use of this boiler water.

The same kind of water is often, no doubt, used by the family in the evening, when hot water is required to mix with wine or spirits, and possibly even with milk for infants. However trifling it may seem to enter into these domestic matters, I know them to be of paramount importance, and the subject could not be fairly exposed without mentioning them. I am not, therefore, afraid of any ridicule which may be attached to thus descending into particulars. But in many cases these boilers are rendered still further unwholesome by containing coils of lead pipe, which are intended to convey hot water to baths, situated above them. These pipes become corroded by the water, as I shall have occasion to show, and the evaporation from the boiler tends to concentrate the poison. There could not, therefore, be well imagined a contrivance which is so adapted for a mischievous use.

The pumps, which supply spring water are generally placed in yards, at some little distance from the house, so that servants, in order to save trouble, or escape rain, are led to avail themselves of the means I have mentioned. In other cases, there are no pumps belonging to the house, so that a man is probably employed to fetch water, as it is wanted, and the supply being contingent on this source, is not always sufficient to meet the exigencies of the household. The water may sometimes be obtained from a proper source, and sometimes from a wrong one, and often it may be got from a mixed source, and hence the mischief may never be fairly discovered, and the consequent disease not amount to a degree sufficient to challenge attention. I am sure many anomalous cases of dyspepsia have such an origin, and the medical man, who should attribute these to their right source, would, I fear, be thought very fanciful, and be often unable to establish the truth of his own position.

Something of the same obscurity may arise from the use of filters. It is true that filters remove the greater portion of the lead from the water, so that it may be drunk with little danger for long periods, if, indeed, it ever produce mischief; but, in addition to the possibility of some filters being imperfect, or out of repair, they do not always get supplied regularly, and the varying wants of families may frequently lead to unfiltered water being used. Hence we have cases of great obscurity, so that it is better not to trust to defences of this kind, unless we are prepared to inspect the matter constantly for ourselves.

After what I have already said, I need scarcely excuse myself for dwelling on such small matters. So much, indeed, am I impressed with the importance of this subject, that I should recommend those who are located in lodging-houses, or who are in the habit of travelling from place to place, to furnish themselves with the means of testing water, that they may make an inquiry, from time to time, into the nature of the water brought to the table. This may, at any rate, be a desirable caution for those who have already suffered from lead colic, or have dyspeptic symptoms for which they cannot find relief, and are ignorant of the cause. I have chosen to speak particularly of these points, because I conceive that if there be any merit in these pages, it is chiefly in the prominence which I have given to matters apparently so trivial.

In the outskirts of large towns, many of the houses, particularly the new ones, have lead pumps; and in watering places, I think, there are often lead pumps, and sometimes a deficiency of pumps altogether; so that soft water is used at the lodging-houses. I have known persons return from watering places with vomiting and griping pains, which may have taken their origin in saturnine contamination. When I was last at Blackpool, I saw many lead pumps, and some of the houses had no pumps whatever. If these places are visited for the benefit of health, it would be well, at least, that they should not be productive of disease.

The sulphuretted hydrogen is the best test for lead, and indeed the only available one for the more minute quantities. It may be diffused in water, and kept in a closely-stoppered bottle; but after a time, the gas is decomposed and sulphur becomes deposited, and the odour of the gas is lost. It is necessary, therefore, that the test should be recently prepared, and that when it is used the peculiar odour should be perceived in it. The precipitate produced is of a brownish colour, and *not* black; indeed, if the precipitate should be black, we may almost suspect that it is owing to the presence of iron. I remember, on one occasion, speaking to a gentleman about the subject of contaminated water, and he proposed that I should examine the water from his own pump. Being himself fond of chemical pursuits, we repaired to his laboratory, and having procured some of the water, passed a stream of sulphuretted hydrogen through it. The water rapidly turned black, like ink, and I was at first disposed to think that this arose from lead, but I had not then leisure to pursue the examination. I was told, afterwards, that there was no lead about the pump, and assured by a respectable chemist that the precipitate was from iron. This I afterwards corroborated by the use of other tests, and by finding the precipitate soluble in muriatic acid. I then made an artificial carbonate of iron by precipitating sulphate of iron with the carbonate of magnesia. Over the surface of the green precipitate which fell, the water became of a faint brownish colour. This I decanted off, and tested with the sulphuretted hydrogen, and it gave a black precipitate similar to what I have described. The iron clay-stone, which, I believe, contains carbonate of iron, will therefore be liable to give a black precipitate with sulphuretted hydrogen, and this must not be mistaken for lead.

I have no pretensions myself to any great amount of chemical knowledge, and, indeed, should always refer to professed chemists if I had any doubt; but in all the cases in which I have suspected lead disease, I have never experienced any difficulty in arriving at a decision. I have not only had the symptoms to guide me, on which I can almost rely by themselves, but optical evidence that the water was contained in lead cisterns, pumps, or pipes; besides the evidence derived from the efficacy of a treatment directed to the lead disorder. But, as the best of all evidences, I have found patients rapidly improve who have followed my advice in giving up the water which was contaminated. At the same time, however, that I do not pretend to any great chemical knowledge, I have found the little I possess, very useful, and generally quite adequate to inquiries such as these. The sulphate of potass and soda, and iodide of potass, &c., mentioned in books as tests for lead, are not delicate enough for lead as it exists in water. The hydrosulphuret of ammonia may do as a rough sort of test, but will not be accurate enough for minute inquiries, and is objectionable on account of its colour; yet, as it is easily procured and carried about, it may be used in some cases with advantage, previous to more accurate inquiries. In choosing the water for the purpose of investigation, it is necessary to observe some rules.

If it be taken from a pump, it should be taken early in the morning, before the pump has been otherwise used, and the first water drawn made the subject of experiment. The reason for this precaution is, obviously, that the water has stood longer in contact with the lead,—a circumstance which makes considerable difference in the contamination. I once visited a family where a female servant had the lead colic. I took some of the water with me, and tested it when I got home. It showed evidences of lead; and the next morning I thought I would repeat the experiment for the family. This I did at their own house; but, to my surprise, the test produced no effect whatever. I was at first at a loss to know the reason; but seeing a carriage standing in the yard, it struck me that the carriage might have been cleaned with water from the same pump. This, I was told, was actually the case. I then desired the family to try the experiment themselves, early the next morning, and I left my test for that purpose. The lady of the house told me on the following day that the trial was attended with the results which I had mentioned. On another occasion, I attended a gentleman who suffered from drinking contaminated water, and who, happening to be a person of observation, immediately perceived the importance of the subject, and aided me in every way in the investigation. He sent me several bottles of water from his pump,—amongst them, one after the pump had been at rest for forty-eight hours, and another after it had been worked for ten minutes previously. The first was strongly contaminated with lead, and the second gave no evidence of it. It is, therefore, as well, when we wish to trace the minuter quantities, to obtain the water for ourselves; or get it procured under the most favorable circumstances. The water, which is contaminated with lead, is not necessarily distinguishable from pure water; so that it must not be supposed that it can always be discovered by the sight.

Soft water, which has stood in a lead cistern, is, however, generally not clear; and if poured into a vessel by the side of pure spring water, the contrast is very apparent. The soft water has the appearance, when held up to the light, of having a small dust-like sediment suspended in it.—There are minute little specks diffused in it, which take off its brilliance, and are, I suppose, in point of fact, small particles of carbonate of lead, for a filter even of paper removes the principal part of the contamination. In other cases, the water is clear when first drawn, as in the instance of pump water, but after some exposure to the air, a white film appears of carbonate of lead. Dr. Christison alludes to a case in which a gentleman discovered the contamination of the water in his dressing-room by seeing a film lining his water-bottle. The gentleman's attention had been attracted to this subject by reading an article in 'Chambers'

Journal.' It is obvious, however, that all deposits are not of lead, and those which take place after boiling water are generally of lime.

With regard to the quantity of lead required to produce the effects of saturnine poisoning, it is altogether impossible to speak,—more particularly as much depends on its cumulative influence, and much also on constitutional peculiarity. It is, perhaps, to be regretted, that Dr. Thomson and Dr. Christison have made some remarks on this question, which, however correct in themselves, may possibly lead to a continuance of the use of lead for holding or conveying water.

It is enough to know that all lead contamination is objectionable; and no degree of contamination is, in my opinion, safe. The colour of the precipitate is to a great extent indicative of the amount of impurity; and I have found it vary from a coffee colour to a pale brownish or yellow tinge, scarcely perceptible. It is as well always to pour out two vessels of water, and, having added the test to one, to compare it with the other, by the aid of transmitted light, and always in the day-time.

But the principal of all points, with respect to the detection of mischief from lead, is a proper knowledge of the symptoms which lead produces; for the ways in which it may be taken into the system are so numerous, that it would be impossible, without this knowledge, to guard against the danger. Besides, if we had no suspicion excited by the nature of the complaint, we should never be led to enter into the inquiry; for chemical investigation must, in the majority of instances, be instigated by a suspicion of the cause. Above all other means, then, of rendering us fully alive to the danger, and making the protection commensurate with the evil, is a proper acquaintance with the disorders produced by lead.

Nor does it seem to me that this knowledge is so present in the minds of the majority of practitioners as it ought to be. I will not suppose that medical men are wanting in an acquaintance with the subject,—it is too much a part of their earliest education to be deficient; but I have said it is not so *present* as it should be,—and I will add, that it is scarcely so extended, as it might with advantage be made. The profession will have to judge me in making these remarks; but I think the honest members of it will not think I am exceeding the truth. I can only say, without arrogating to myself superior discrimination, that circumstances have happened to press this subject on my own mind. The inquiries which I have made, respecting the effects of water contaminated with lead on the health of my patients, have been far from personally advantageous to me in the practice of my profession. In abandoning the usual routine method of practice, I have seemed to many, no doubt, inquisitorial or fanciful, or have appeared embarrassed and doubtful, in cases which to others might be deemed sufficiently simple. Some persons have actually expressed themselves affronted that I should suppose they were not sufficiently careful as to the water they were in the habit of drinking. Besides, more time has been given to inquiries respecting the nature of water than it is customary to bestow in the usual visitations of the sick. Again, in seeking to enlarge our knowledge on the effects of contaminated water, I have been wishful to ascertain if any symptoms not usually ascribed to this source could be found referable to it; and, in keeping my mind open to this possibility, I have necessarily had to suspend my judgment where it would have been easy to decide if everything might have been determined by the observations of previous writers. It must be confessed also, and chiefly perhaps from this latter reason, that I have sometimes felt and expressed suspicions as to the contamination of water, which a careful inquiry was unable to confirm. It will be thus apparent, I think, that minute investigations of this sort are not likely to be attended with much credit, either in the eyes of the public or of the profession; and, if one were merely to study reputation, one would rather wait for marked cases than anticipate discovery by following the subject into its finer ramifications. Being myself, however, fairly impressed with the magnitude of the evil, I do not think I ought to be influenced by any considerations of personal advantage.

Though I value very highly the opinion of my professional brethren, and, in the treatment of many complaints, have been very desirous of associating myself with others, I cannot say that in these investigations I have been much forwarded by professional consultations. The inquiry is one which can only be pursued by a careful and detailed examination of matters which have been made so little the subject of ordinary medical attention, that few are prepared to enter on the matter with the requisite patience and impartiality; and many, no doubt, can scarcely afford the time which is in reality necessary.

In addition to the trouble of examining into the nature of water, and the apparent irregularity of directing inquiries into matters of this nature, I have found it difficult to convince patients of the danger of using the contaminated water. In many instances an unwilling assent has been the only reward of considerable labour; sometimes, a smile of incredulity, and, at other times, contradiction has been openly expressed where there was no possibility of doubt. In reality, it must be allowed that there are many circumstances which render it difficult for non-professional persons to understand the true bearings of the subject. The patient may have taken the contaminated water for a long period, and, after much imperfect health, may have suddenly become ill; and this illness may seem to be immediately attributable to some ordinary indiscretion in diet. He may further be the only one affected, out of a family who reside in the same dwelling, and who may be said, in general language, to be living under the same circumstances, and partaking of the same water. These difficulties can only be cleared up by a knowledge which many do not possess.—The poison of lead is what is called a *cumulative* poison, and may be taken for a long period, in small quantities, before any mischief is experienced. This is not the case with all poisonous substances; for some may be taken regularly without any other bad effects than the repetition of a hurtful impression which must gradually impair the health; but, in the instance of cumulative poisons, the effect continues for a considerable period after the administration of each dose, so that a period comes when the system is overwhelmed with it. But this event is brought about in so gradual and insidious a manner, that the change is scarcely perceived, and the full amount of the evil is only made evident by some cause which calls for the unusual efforts of the organ which is affected.

There is another point which tends to obscure the subject, namely, the *elective* action of the poison. From many who are placed in parallel circumstances, one in particular seems to be chosen. This arises in a great measure from peculiarity of constitution, which renders one person more susceptible than another of certain impressions. Medical men are accustomed to meet with great differences in this respect, and they have employed the term *idiosyncracy* to express this individuality of constitutional nature. Idiosyncracy has much to do with the rapidity with which lead produces its effect; and it is to be borne in mind that the first person prominently affected, will, for the time being, seem the only person that is affected at all.—Habits also must have much to do in determining the election of the poison.

Some persons drink little water, and are from home the greater part of the day. Children have frequently milk to drink; many persons take ale and porter, or wine. Where the family *do* drink water, it may be persumed that it is more frequently filtered for the master and mistress of the family, than for the domestics. Accordingly I have found that a great number of cases of lead-disease have arisen amongst servants. But a still more frequent reason that the servants are the chief sufferers is, that they are more in the habit of drinking soft water, in the manner I have already named. It will be evident, then, that the habits as well as the idiosyncracy of the patient have much to do in determining the election of the poison.

A complaint, which is so gradually induced, is necessarily very insidious in its progress;—when day after day produces no perceptible effect, it is difficult to tell at what period the morbid influence may be said to have become apparent. In fact, the patient loses his health in such gentle gradations that he continues to think himself well, or rather loses that just appreciation of health which would attend the more speedy transitions. He considers himself dyspeptic, is troubled with constipation, becomes slightly emaciated, perceives his respiration to be difficult, and feels to have lost his usual elasticity of mind and of body. Pain now begins to be experienced in the epigastrium; the constipation is more troublesome; and aching sensations are felt in the limbs. The complexion gradually assumes a dirty yellow cast, and the margin of the gums has sometimes a bluish appearance, or borders the teeth in places with a deep blue line. This state may be, in part, and for a time, arrested by purgatives and medicines, but especially, and for obvious reasons, by a temporary change of place. The sufferer conceives that his residence is unhealthy, and without suspecting the true cause, blames various circumstances in his locality or dwelling. The muscles now begin to lose their accustomed strength; the patient walks badly, holds his pen with less steadiness, and vomits apparently without adequate cause;—after a protracted period of ill health, to which he is become familiar, and perhaps to some extent indifferent, he suddenly becomes seized with a griping pain in the stomach. He takes aperient medicine, but it is vomited; he repeats the dose, but without effect: the pain goes on increasing, and at length becomes intolerable and unintermitting; medicine after medicine is rejected. He tosses himself about in extreme and increasing distress; now vomiting green porraceous matter, and now vainly trying by pressure and friction to mitigate his suffering. If this state be not relieved by timely and judicious assistance, convulsions arise and insensibility comes on, and even death may follow. By this time he will be found to have acquired a dirty yellow tinge, and to have a wretched look with some emaciation, and a partially paralysed and wasted state of the muscles. He has probably walked with a shuffling gait, and felt his mind give way, and even his words falter.

But this is not the invariable train of symptoms which attend the slow poisoning of lead; but it is one which is the most notable, and, so to say, the type of the disease. In some cases rheumatic feelings are prominently complained of, and in others the paralytic affection is more pronounced than the rest. Again, extraordinary nervous sensations have marked the beginning of the disorder; but these various symptoms will come before us in succession as we proceed with the subject.

In describing a complaint, we must portray the more common phenomena, and of those which relate to saturnine poisoning, the most characteristic are, constipation, abdominal pain, and vomiting. If I must add others, they are those of pain in the lower part of the spine, and a failure in the muscular power. But no symptom can be well interpreted without reference to the rest, and it is the sum of the symptoms which makes up the disease. Sometimes the complaint is relieved for a time without its being properly understood, and then the attacks are repeated after intervals of imperfect health of greater or of less duration.

The protracted suffering continues, however, until the health is irrevocably injured. In some of these cases the original symptoms have given place to others, and it has seemed to me that a kind of tolerance has been acquired, more dangerous to the patient as the urgency is the less. Constipation has been succeeded by a sort of chronic dysentery, and the colic and vomiting have been replaced by palsy and rheumatism. The complaint no longer makes those loud demands for relief which it was accustomed to do, but is no less terrible in reality; and the sufferer, at last, dies of epilepsy, or sinks into the grave in a manner that is never understood, and another victim follows before attention is aroused.

This chronic state of disease is the most important, because it is the least likely to arrest attention, and is a form of complaint peculiarly liable to arise from the more subtle manner in which lead may be taken in contaminated water. But I shall shortly take an opportunity of pointing out that the chronic form of disease is not unfrequent to the artisans who are employed in the manufactures of lead.

In describing this slow form of lead affection, I have, perhaps, not sufficiently remarked upon the pain which is experienced in the lower part of the spine. I have even known this symptom to be the most insisted on, and made a principal subject of complaint. It is generally, however, aecompanied with pain in the pit of the stomach, and the other derangements which I have mentioned. This pain in the lower part of the spine is a peculiar aching sensation radiating into the limbs, and may be falsely conceived in the female, in whom it, perhaps, chiefly occurs, to be an indication of uterine disturbance.

It is natural to suppose that the name *Rachialgia*, which was given by Astruc to the affection produced by lead, was particularly derived from this single symptom, (ραχις, the spine, and αλγος, pain,) but I find that term is more generally ascribed to a theory which referred the whole malady to a derangement of the nervès.

Bouillaud says,[1] "Astruc pensait que les coliques dont il s'agit, n'avaient point leur siége dans le ventre, mais bien dans les nerfs qui tirent leur origine de la moelle épinière, et de là le nom de *rachialgie*, qu'il imposa à la colique de plomb. Cette opinion offre quelque chose d'assez vraisemblable; il faut convenir au moins que jusqu'ici, les nevralgies sont entre toutes les maladies, celles dont la colique de plomb parait se rapprocher le plus."

I have stated that the chronic form of

[1] Dict. de Médecine.

disease is not peculiar to the drinking of contaminated water, and is, indeed, common to those employed habitually in the arts where lead is concerned. It is incidentally alluded to by that very able and excellent writer Sir George Baker, in his admirable and highly philosophical inquiry into the origin of the Devonshire Colic. I shall gladly avail myself of a quotation from his writings, which I have everywhere found most useful for reference and consultation. In speaking of the disorder as it affects the artificers of lead, he says: "But there is a chronic species of this malady still more formidable in its effects, which not unfrequently occurs, and to which, as far as I have observed, persons of thin, tender, irritable habits are particularly subject. The first beginnings of it are slight, and generally are, therefore, not much regarded. In this state it is sometimes referred to causes which do not exist; and opposed by medicines, which, perhaps, tend only to co-operate with the disease. In the mean time, it steals on by slow progression; each successive paroxysm becomes more severe than the former; and the patient is at length reduced to the most deplorable state of infirmity;—his muscles waste, his limbs are contracted, his respiration is difficult, and after having a long time dragged on a most miserable existence, he dies, either convulsed, or apoplectic."[1]

My friend, Dr. Norris of Stourbridge, has recently directed attention to the same subject in the pages of the 'Lancet.' He properly insists on the importance of attending to the more slow and insidious forms of the disease in the artificers of lead. He describes the mental and physical depression which ensues, where,—

> "Yellow sickness sits cavern'd in the hollow eye."[2]

It is curious that Dr. Norris, after giving

[1] Med.-Chir. Trans., vol. i, p. 258.
[2] Lancet, vol. lxii, p. 6, 1852.

much attention to these matters, was yet unaware, for many years, that he was himself the subject of lead disease from contaminated water. It is interesting to notice this, as a proof how easily that source of the poison may elude observation. I shall relate his case before I conclude my remarks.

Thus, then, we have an almost numistakable assemblage of symptoms, an assemblage which should, at any rate, always raise the inquiry,—can the patient be suffering from the poison of lead?

We have constipation, debility, an harassing pain in the stomach and back, and difficult respiration, progressive wasting and palsy, a sallow countenance, and probably a blue mark on the gums. If we have, in addition, attacks of violent and unmitigated colic, and vomiting, we can scarcely avoid the conclusion that the disorder is produced by lead. But these attacks may have passed away, and a state of broken health may remain, the nature of which may elude the routine method of inquiry, into which even able and humane physicians must necessarily be led by the number of their engagements.

I shall proceed, however, to examine the symptoms individually,—and here, I may remark, that I have found great assistance from the perusal of writers who have treated on the effects of lead in the arts. They describe the same morbid phenomena which arise from the more gradual poisoning by contaminated water, allowing only for the greater rapidity or urgency of the result. I may especially mention the able works of Mérat and Tanquerel Desplanches, the latter, indeed, leaving little to be accomplished by succeeding writers. With great opportunities for observation, he has written with all that fulness and diligence of research which distinguish our continental friends.

Mérat, as an earlier author, had perhaps equal merit in what he accomplished, but the work of Tanquerel Desplanches is more extended, and consequently more complete. I have adopted some of the terms made use of by Tanquerel, and I have done so with some reluctance, as I have no great ambition to multiply technical phraseology. I find, however, that there are no words in general use which can, with propriety, be employed to express the ideas that it was necessary to set forth.

A very interesting circumstance was discovered, somewhat accidentally, by Dr. Burton, in respect to the effects of lead on the gums. Dr. Burton first directed his attention to this subject in the year 1834. It having been supposed that a patient under Dr. Roots, his late colleague at St. Thomas's Hospital, had been salivated by the internal use of lead, he was induced to examine the mouths of the patients admitted into his own wards; "who had been exposed to the action of lead in the course of their usual avocations; and of those who had swallowed the acetate of lead medicinally." From this inquiry he was led to conclude that salivation was by no means a frequent occurrence; but he noticed, in most cases, a peculiar blue discoloration of the gums. The margins of the gums, at the borders of the teeth, were marked by a dark, narrow, blue line, and this was attended with no fetor of the breath. The discoloration was very permanent, and he remarked that it remained, and even became more visible, after death.

Dr. Burton considered himself the first to point out this symptom, and he properly attached considerable value to it. Authors seem indeed to have observed a bluish cast of the saliva, though they do not mention the condition of the gums. Thus Dr. Christison, in his 'Treatise on Poisons,' (1829,) says, speaking of the effects of lead, "the saliva is increased in quantity, and *bluish* in colour;" and Dr. A. T. Thompson states,[1] "the saliva assumes a bluish colour." The blue colour of the gums is, however, much more palpable than that of the saliva; and Dr. Burton's paper, which will be found in the 23d vol. of the 'Med.-Chir. Transactions,' is a really valuable contribution to science, and a very ably-written paper. The blue appearance is not always so well marked as Dr. Burton describes it, and is often absent altogether, even when the patient is decidedly affected with lead. When it *is* found, however, it is a most important aid in diagnosis; and, indeed, in most, if not all the cases in which this appearance *cannot* be traced to lead, the insidious introduction of lead may yet be suspected. Instead of showing itself in a deep blue line, as it frequently does, it sometimes shows itself in a soft blue discoloration, gradually shading deeper towards the teeth.

[1] Therapeutics, vol. ii, p. 64.

It is generally most visible on one or two of the incisor or canine teeth, and sometimes a slate-coloured hue has been found also in the inside of the mouth. Though we must not then rely on the absence of this sign, as a sure indication that there is no lead affection, we may feel very strong corroboration of our belief in the existence of such disorder (if not absolute certainty) where we *do* find it;—an examination of the gums should, therefore, never be neglected. Nay, it may be of assistance in inquiries, where doubt may exist, to examine the mouths of those in the same household with the patient; to ascertain if any other member of the family has this peculiarity, for the colour sometimes exists before any striking evidence of general derangement.

Dr. Burton relates two very interesting cases where the patients had the blue discoloration of the gums and other symptoms of lead disease; but he was not able at the time to trace the complaint to its proper source. He mentions, however, that these patients were in the habit of drinking water from a leaden cistern, which he probably was not fully aware would be a very sufficient cause.—The first case was that of a carpenter. He had never worked in lead, nor was there any suspicion of his having been exposed to its influence. About four years before he was admitted to the hospital, (St. Thomas's,) he had suffered a severe illness, which was followed by a palsy of his fingers. He became languid and feeble; his appetite failed, and his limbs felt heavy, and he experienced a pain in his stomach, which extended to the breast, the shoulders, and the arms. His bowels became constipated, and vomiting occurred;—his nights were spent without sleep;—his countenance was pale, and there was a trembling noticed in his hands;—the gums had the blue border. —The second instance was that of a cordwainer, who had resided in the country previous to his admission into the hospital. He had been confined to bed seventeen times with colic, but he was free from paralysis. During these attacks he had endured violent pain in the bowels, frequent vomiting, and obstinate constipation and loss of rest. He was thin, and his complexion sallow; the gums were marked by the blue discoloration.

No doubt, in cases where lead is immediately brought in contact with the gums in a state of dust or vapour, the blue border will be the most apparent; but it is a mistake to suppose that the discoloration may not arise from less direct causes. The remarks made by Brachet, in his recent work on the 'Colique de Plomb,' therefore require modification. He says on this subject—"Aussi la plupart des observations qui en font mention, ont été recueillies sur les ouvriers qui travaillent dans les fabriques de céruse; tandis que le plomb qui n'agira que sur la peau ou *dans les voies digestives*, ne produira guère ce phénomène."[1]—He properly, however, allows that in this opinion he may be wrong, as he undoubtedly is.

Tanquerel Desplanches also, in my opinion, ascribes too much to the contact of particles of lead in producing this effect. I have, over and over again, found the blue margin in persons who have taken contaminated water; and it can hardly be supposed that the effect is occasioned by the mere passage of the water over the gums or between the teeth. "La teinte des gencives," says Tanquerel, "et des dents que nous venons de décrire nous ne l'avons jamais observée, que chez les individus dont la membrane muqueuse buccale, s'est trouvé en contact avec des particules de plomb."[2]

A very unnecessary, and indeed hurtful, practice seems tacitly recommended by this author, namely, that of *brushing the teeth*

[1] P. 142. [2] 'Traité des Maladies de Plomb,' vol. i, p. 8.

frequently and for many days with water acidified with the sulphuric and muriatic acids.—Common cleanliness seems to me all that is required when the cause is abandoned.

Besides the blue discoloration, the gums sometimes present a dark brown or reddish line; but this is less to be relied on, and may be more likely to be dependent on common causes. The gums which have assumed the blue colour are also wasted. The blue discoloration has, I think, been attributed to the chemical agency of the tartar which collects in the mouth. I believe that I have noticed the mark to be the strongest in cases where the tartar was present, but I have seen it also exist where there was none. It is easy to suppose that in whatever form sulphur may exist, whether in the saliva itself, or the salts which it deposits, it may serve as a natural test for the presence of lead.

The length of time necessary for the production of the blue line differs according to the quantity of lead taken. Dr. Burton says—"Mr. Moyle, of Chacewater, produced the discoloration in twenty-four hours, by giving four doses of five grains each of the acetate of lead every six hours;" and "I think (he adds) that in cases of poisoning from the irritant effects of large doses of the soluble salts of lead, similar to those described by Dr. Christison, the discoloration would be obvious on the gums in five hours after swallowing the salts, although the time required in several cases under my own care was much longer, in which large medicinal doses of the acetate were given frequently in twenty-four hours."[1]

Perhaps no single symptom produced by the poison of lead is so well known as that of colic. Many persons, who are not conversant with its other effects, are still familiar with the names of the Painters' Colic and

[1] Med.-Chir. Trans., vol. xxiii, p. 78.

the Colic of Poitou. But this colic does not in reality arise until the patient has been suffering some time from the poison, though his attention may not probably have been arrested by his previous indisposition. The bowels will be found to have become gradually constipated, but not entirely obstructed; pains have been felt in the pit of the stomach or about the navel, but they have not been such as to excite any partienlar anxiety. At length, the pain becomes exceedingly troublesome, and such as can scarcely be endured.[1] Medicine is taken, but no action is produced on the bowels; it is repeated, and vomiting arises. The pain becomes at length intolerable; more medicine is taken, and more vomiting produced. It is now almost continuous, but yet aggra-

[1] Among the German miners the name of "Hütten Katze," or cat of the foundry, has been used to describe the torments of lead colic, which are thought to resemble the sensation of the intestines being torn to pieces by a cat.—*Dr. Alderson's Lumleian Lectures.* ('Lancet,' 1852, p. 97.)

vated by movements. The patient involuntarily presses his hand over his stomach or bowels, or turns uneasily to lie on his abdomen. All fluids are rejected, and the contents thrown from the stomach are green and acid; yet the vomiting gives no relief. The sufferer groans in unceasing and intolerable pain. The patient generally bears pressure well, if gently and steadily made; but this is not always the case, for the abdomen is sometimes rendered extremely tender by the retching and vomiting which have occurred. It is commonly said that the abdomen is shrunk and, as it is called, *retracted;* but this is not to be considered a condition universally found; on the contrary, it is sometimes full, and frequently natural in appearance.

Dr. Warren, who has written well upon this complaint, observes—"It is remarkable that two distant parts of the body are seldom affected at the same time. If the pain is in the stomach, the lower bowels are generally easy, the external muscles always; if the external muscles are in pain, the stomach and bowels are perfectly free, and the patient is apt to imagine that his disorder is gone off, or converted into another; but he is soon undeceived, and at the end of two or three hours feels his pain returning, with all its violence, to its old seat, the region of the navel or the pit of the stomach. When the pain is seated near the navel, and the patient complains that he feels as if he was being bored through with an instrument, the abdominal muscles are sometimes knotted, sometimes painfully retracted, with all the contents of the abdomen, towards the spine. In whatever part of the bowel the pain is seated, there is frequently a very cousiderable fulness and tension of the abdomen. The pain does not, as in some colics, abate and increase several times in a few minutes, but generally observes the same tenor for several hours together; sometimes it has exacerbations, and then it admits of truces for two or three hours.[1] Along with this colic, a contraction of the *sphincter ani* is noticed, so that it is with difficulty that a clyster can be administered; and the urine is passed with difficulty. The pulse is not usually affected, though it may become so if the complaint be long without relief. The urine is various in appearance, and sometimes deposits a lateritious sediment. The alvine evacuations are generally dark, and what is called scybalous. Constipation is a common attendant on the colic, but there are cases in which the bowels are relaxed. The constipatiou generally bears a relation to the pain which is experienced.—It is, then, to be borne in mind that, whilst these things differ in particular instances, constipation is, for the most part, a very leading symptom in the affections of lead.—We must be pre-

[1] Med.-Chir. Trans., vol. ii, p. 70.

pared, however, occasionally to meet with varieties, and we should not refuse to admit the exceptions. Tanquerel Desplanches says that out of 1217 patients, 1140 had constipation, 33 had a natural state of the bowels, 25 were purged during the first two days of their illness, and 19 were so during the whole period of the affection.[1] The occasional effect of the poison in relaxing the bowels was noticed very long ago.

Galen remarked that diarrhœa arose from drinking water which had acquired a saturnine impregnation.

Citois observes of the colic of Poitou, that it was often attended "per initia præsertim, cum alvi frequenti, sed non ita copioso, fluore, sæpius cum ejusdem adstrictione." M. Doazam, who writes on the same disease in the 'Journal de Médecine' for October, 1760, remarks—"Il en est plusieurs, qui non seulement n'ont point épreuvé

[1] Vol. i, p. 203.

de constipation, mais même qui se sont plaints d'un flux de ventre."[1]

The duration of the colic varies; it may last many days, subsiding and returning, and much must depend on the manner in which it is combated. If it be treated with proper and decisive means, it does not generally continue long, and the pain is commonly relieved when the bowels have been fairly purged.

The poison of lead not only produces pains in the bowels, but also in the limbs. These pains are generally considered as the result of rheumatism, although they differ essentially from that complaint in many particulars. The pains are often very intolerable in their nature, and have been variously described, according to the fancy of the sufferer; they are said to be *boring*, tearing, or burning sensations; sensations as if teeth were gnawing to the bones.

[1] Med.-Chir. Trans., vol. i, p. 238.

They become worse in the night than in the day. Unlike rheumatism, they are not accompanied with a disturbance of the pulse, nor are they productive of swelling nor redness, nor of tenderness to the touch. They thus differ markedly from acute rheumatism, but still they are often described and considered as such. In some cases excessive sensibility attends these sensations, so exalted, indeed, that a slight wafting of the air is productive of acute pain. There are certain parts of the body which seem more frequently the subjects of the disorder, particularly the flexures of the joints, so that painful contractions come on with the more violent pains. The muscles may be seen to gather in lumps, and the patient leaps from his bed to stretch his limbs. The legs more frequently suffer than the arms. I have often heard patients, particularly females, complain of pain in the lower part of the spine, and this, I imagine to be, a common seat of the affection. The pains are aggravated by movement, and yet the patient cannot remain still, as he would be glad to do, in acute rheumatism. Much, therefore, as they resemble rheumatism, they have, as I have remarked, several characteristic differences:—there is the violence of the pain, notwithstanding the freedom from redness, from swelling, and from fever;—the restlessness of the patient, notwithstanding his suffering,—and together with these, there are contractions of the limbs. But we have, perhaps, better indications in the accompanying or preceding colic, in the discoloured gums, in the sallow complexion, and in the wasting and debility of the muscles. It is true that perspirations accompany these pains as they do those of ordinary rheumatism.

Almost equally familiar with the colic, is the Palsy produced by lead. The dropping of the wrists and the wasting of the muscles in painters and others, who are employed in the trades where lead is used, have become subjects of general remark. The palsy of lead is mostly preceded by the colic, and the latter furnishes us, therefore, with much insight into the nature of the former. From some cause or other, which is perhaps not well understood, the extensor muscles of the body are especially liable to suffer, and this often in a very partial manner. Hence arise the contractions of the joints, which are so remarkable in this species of palsy.

The palsy is said more generally to affect the upper extremities, and a wasting of the fleshy part of the thumb has been particularly noticed. This may, in some degree perhaps, be ascribed to the more frequent local application of lead to the arms and hands than the legs, and is, at least, not an invariable form of the affection. The palsy of lead is accompanied with the racking pains in the limbs, which have been noticed, and with painful contractions, more observed in the night thàn the day.

Colic does not exist as a necessary part of the complaint, nor has it invariably preceded it. The palsy of lead seems partieularly to affect certain muscles,—and the pains which accompany it especially select the calves of the legs, and the soles and margins of the feet. The muscles of the chest and arms are also often affected, and the voice is sometimes altered and weakened by the same influence. A paralysis of the intercostal muscles, and of those which affect the respiration, is probably a chief cause of the difficulty which is felt in breathing. The patient has also often a stammering in his speech, likewise ascribable to the failure of the implicated muscles.

The palsy of lead generally begins gradually, in a sort of numbness (*engourdissement*) and trembling, with an uncertainty or incapability of directing the movements of the body. It is not easy to say why some persons should be more liable than others to suffer from the palsy; but, whilst many are tortured with frequent attacks of colic, a few are attacked with an early paralysis.[1] There are varieties also in the manner in which it occurs. The upper extremities are most frequently affected, but sometimes the lower are the only parts to suffer. It may be sufficient to know that diversities may be expected, and sometimes there is a sort of

[1] Dr. Alderson suggests that paralysis may be more likely to arise from the introduction of lead through the respiratory passages in fumes and dust, as being more speedy,—and colic from its reception into the alimentary canal. In illustration, he remarks on the different effects produced by mercury when inhaled by water-gilders, and when taken as a medicine. In the former case it produces tremblings, which are unknown in the latter. He thinks it probable that the dust of carbonate of lead, which is often floating on the atmosphere of manufactories where lead is used, may be rendered soluble to the respiratory organs by the extra carbonic acid gas evolved by the lungs. (See the Lumleian Lectures' delivered at the Royal College of Physicians, 1852.)

isolation in the peculiar muscles which are concerned.

Where palsy has once occurred from this cause, a repetition of the attack is easily produced, and hence the importance of a rigid avoidance of all circumstances which expose the sufferer to the agency of lead. If the recovery be not complete, it is manifest that little is wanting to renew the disorder; and even where no such indication remains, there is yet a certain proneness in the system to fall into a condition from which it has been but recently emancipated. Where persons have suffered from drinking contaminated water, and have received benefit by a temporary absence from home, they have commonly experienced, on their return, a speedy aggravation of the malady. This is noticed by almost all writers, and hence the natural conclusion, that a change of air was the real source of the improvement.

When the paralysis which results from

lead is very complete, the state of wretchedness is extreme. The picture has been so graphically portrayed by Citois, that I cannot refrain from quoting it.

"Per vicos, veluti larvæ, aut arte progredientes statuæ, pallidi, squallidi, macilenti conspiciuntur, manibus incurvis et suo pondere pendulis, nec nisi arte ad os et cæteras supernas partes sublatis ac pedibus non suis, sed crurum musculis ad ridiculum, ni miserandum, incessum compositis, voce clangosa et strepera."[1]

Through the villages, they walked like ghosts, or statues, moving by art,—pale, squalid, wasted,—with their hands curved, and hanging by their own weight, and as if attached only by art to the bones and upper parts,—and with feet alien to their bodies, reduced to a step that would be ridiculous, if it were not miserable; there voices clanging and streperous.

[1] Med.-Chir. Trans., vol. i, p. 199.

Dr. Alderson relates an interesting case of paralysis which arose from the drinking of rain water from a lead cistern. It is contained in the paper to which I have already made reference in the 'Medico-Chirurgical Transactions.' In the year 1837, Dr. Alderson was requested by Mr. Craven to visit with him a Mr. Thackray, who was 63 years of age. He found his patient labouring under paralysis of the upper extremities, the hands being powerless by the side, and partial paralysis of the lower extremities;—nor could he raise himself from his chair without assistance. When he walked to his bedroom, he required two servants to walk by his sides, for his knees bent under him, and his gait was tottering. His voice was altered, and his countenance blanched, but his mind was not impaired, and yet he shed tears on the slightest occasion, as we find to be the case in the paralysis from other causes. Dr. Alderson found that his patient had constipation of the bowels, which could not be relieved without very powerful medicine, and he learned from Mr. Craven, that about eighteen months previously, Mr. Thackray had had an epileptic seizure, in which he had fallen out of bed, and dislocated his shoulder. It was further stated that the sister of Mr. Thackray's late wife, who lived in the house with him, and had suffered from a long period of illness, had, about twelve months previously, become similarly paralytic, and died without the cause being properly understood.

The servants had been more or less tormented with colicky pain, but not having resided so long in the house, suffered, consequently, in a minor degree. It had also been remarked, that when Mrs. Martin (Mr. Thackray's sister-in-law) went into Lincolnshire to her native air, she recovered wonderfully from her paralytic symptoms,—but they returned when she came back to Hull.

These circumstances led to an inquiry which resulted in the discovery, that the water used by the family was contaminated with lead. It was rain water collected from the roof of the house, and received into a leaden cistern. It was filtered for use, and had a sweetish taste, which had been often remarked by the servants.

Mr. Pearsall, an able chemist, who adds a note to Dr. Alderson's paper, examined the water; and he remarks on the necessity of examining the deposits at the bottom of suspected water, for he found that, after the cistern water had been agitated, the lead was no longer discoverable in the water, but the black sediment, when boiled with pure nitric acid, and the excess of acid driven off, gave evidence of strong saturnine impregnation.—I have myself sometimes been disappointed in detecting lead in water, when I anticipated discovering it; for on some occasions, I have found that even soft water obtained from boilers communicating with lead cisterns, has suffered no change from the usual reagents for lead:—probably an abler chemist than myself might have been more successful in the discovery.

Sometimes, but less frequently, there is a paralysis of sensibility, along with a loss of motion, or even independent of it. A sort of numbness is experienced either throughout the affected limb, or on the surface of the skin, and may, like the other paralysis, be very partial in its extent.

Dr. Alderson, in the paper recently mentioned, has furnished us with two very interesting cases, in which there was a paralysis of the nerves of vision. The first case was that of Elizabeth Clayton, a young woman of 25, who was a patient of the General Infirmary at Hull.—She had worked seven or eight years in the lead-works, and had never before been attacked with paralysis. Her hands first became palsied, and in about three weeks afterwards the sight became affected, and eventually she became quite blind. The legs were also paralysed, but she scarcely knew when or how they became affected.

The next case was that of a young woman of the age of 18, who was also admitted to the Infirmary. She had worked only nine months at the lead-works, but yet had suffered frequently from the colic. In addition to paralysis of the hands, she had complete loss of sight. Both these cases were eventually cured; and Dr. Alderson found advantage, in addition to the use of purgatives, from the application of bandages to the eyes, so as to exclude the light. This plan he was induced to make use of by reflecting on the plan, suggested by Dr. Pemberton, of relieving the extensors of the arms by the employment of splints,—and supposing a sort of analogous relief might be afforded to the nerves of sight by a temporary suspension of their functions. The idea was as ingenious as it was successful.

Dr. Alderson seems to have met with other cases, which he does not think it necessary to detail.

Cases are also related by Tanquerel Desplanches as occurring in the arts; and he makes one observation, which is interesting both in relation to this, and other forms of lead paralysis, and which serves to show that recovery is often only imperfect when it seems to be nearly complete:—"Une fois nous avons vu un malade, à peine guéri d'amaurose saturnine, en être de nouveau frappé, sans s'être exposé depuis la guérison au contact du plomb. Un autre de nos malades depuis plusieurs années n'était plus en contact avec le plomb, et cependant il fut de nouveau atteint d'amaurose, de paralysie des membranes supérieurs, de colique, et d'encephalopathie saturnines."[1]

[1] Vol. ii, p. 215.

The amaurosis from lead will occasionally arise very suddenly. Felix Plater, a physician of the sixteenth century, relates the case of a woman who, in the midst of a violent colic, was suddenly seized with convulsions and a blindness so complete, that she could not see the flame of a candle placed before her eyes; at the end of three days she recovered her sight. Some years after, she had a new attack of colic and of blindness, from which she also recovered. The attacks, however, recurred again almost every year, and in the end brought her to the grave.

Deafness may in like manner arise. I once attended a servant-boy with lead colic, who complained of deafness after the attack, as well as of rheumatic feelings, both of which seemed to me to be dependent on the same cause, and they disappeared together. Deafness is not, however, so common as amaurosis, and Tanquerel Desplanches seems to doubt whether it be in reality produced by lead.

"Les auteurs ont parlé d'une manière vague de la surdité produite par le plomb, sans en raporter une seule observation authentique." It seems to me, however, so probable that the sense of hearing may be paralysed by lead, when it is confessedly admitted that the sight and feeling are so, that I do not see any sufficient reason to doubt the cases which are ascribed to this cause.

Besides these paralytic affections, Epilepsy, Delirium, and Coma may arise. The colic may suddenly cease, and the fearful truce be interrupted by an attack of convulsions still more terrible. There is something characteristic in the cerebral disturbance which arises from lead. It seems to partake of the wildness and uncertainty which distinguish the operation of a poison. The delirium may be gentle or fierce, and the epilepsy may pass by quick transitions into coma, which shall again alternate with excitement, in a manner little explicable without a true knowledge of the cause.

The symptoms are altogether less permanent and more capricious in their character than when they arise from ordinary cerebral disturbance; but a great deal of light is shed upon these affections by considering the series of morbid phenomena which have preceded them. If there have been colic or paralysis, and tearing pains, or other indications of the saturnine influence, then there can be little doubt as to the nature of the malady. Yet, it is to be borne in mind, that the cerebral symptoms may be the first, and may be sudden in their invasion; but they do not pass through the regular gradations which distinguish inflammatory lesions. The period of excitement does not pass into one of prostration, but coma and excitement seem to give place to each other; and the physical force seems to be preserved in a manner which could not be maintained if the symptoms were dependent on progressive changes in the brain. Here, too, as in most other cases, the pulse will be consulted with advantage. The pulse is not accelerated by the poison of lead, and, if it be rendered rapid by convulsions, it will be found to subside again after their cessation. Nor will the pulse be found rapid at the commencement of the cerebral disturbance, as we should expect would be the case, if it arose from an inflammatory derangement. Where delirium arises, it is a changeable delirium, passing from one form of disorder to another, until an abrupt attack of epilepsy or a sudden coma interrupts its progress.

There is something in all this which reminds us of hysteric caprice; but we are dealing with a more fearful complaint than hysteria, and the result may be a fatal catastrophe. As the various forms of disorder break in upon us unexpectedly, we are kept in alarm as to what may next arise, and we can only assure the friends of the danger and uncertainty of the complaint. The coma, which succeeds the epilepsy of lead, does not pass off so rapidly as the ordinary stupor which follows an epileptic fit. It may last many hours,—it may continue many days. The intellect does not recover readily from the attack; and even after the patient appears to have regained his reason, he will be found for a cousiderable period to be still under the influence of the poison,—in a sort of sub-delirium, which requires some discrimination.

Probably the cerebral affection, which arises from lead, may be thought to have some resemblance to the delirium tremens; but it is not very likely to be confounded with it, for some of the many peculiarities which we have noticed in the maladies produced by lead, will generally be recognised; and it is, in most cases, easy to learn something of the history of cases of the delirium tremens. Coma also generally forms a part of the disturbance produced by lead, and gives place to delirium or epilepsy, in a manner peculiar to saturnine disease. It is only, therefore, in case of complications, that the attentive and instructed practitioner is likely to feel embarrassed by the "*encépha-lopathie saturnine.*"

When the fits of epilepsy are frequent, and are united with coma and delirium, or the patient occupies the intervals with an unceasing prattle, it may be supposed that the danger is extreme. In these cases it is not to be presumed that the other effects of lead poison are absent, for the patient will often show indications of violent colic. Even during a state of unconsciousness, or partial consciousness, he will be observed to place his hand over the abdomen, and rub his stomach, or toss uneasily from side to side, in a manner which indicates pain. His countenance also will show the yellow, waxlike appearance which has been noticed as a symptom of lead disease.

Mérat speaks of the termination of frequent attacks of lead colic in a kind of general *cachexy*. I believe a general cachetic condition may arise from the injury sustained by drinking contaminated water. If the complaint be not properly understood, and the treatment be undertaken without the cause being removed, the patient will fall into a condition in which it is at last almost impossible to recognise the original disorder. The patient may even continue to suffer after he is removed from the source of his distemper, so that no guide remains to indicate its nature. He may have left his abode, and be translated to another town or neighbourhood. He will say that his health is broken, and that he has now no more faith in physic, of which, probably, he has only had too much, (the *bane* having been with him as well as the antidote.) He has great debility, a trembling, unsteady carriage of his body, a tottering in his walk, and a pale and sallow complexion. He has wandering pains in his limbs or back, and, probably, is much oppressed with indigestion, and has a constipation of the bowels. This state of body admits of some amendment, but, in all probability, the system will be found permanently impaired. Such, then, are the results of a disease, the source of which is often little suspected.

It may be imagined, from what I have said, that so many general symptoms are attributed to the poison of lead, that it is almost impossible to determine when the lead affection is really present. It must be observed, then, that the more important and characteristic symptoms are in themselves sufficiently distinctive; and that the rest have only a value when found in combination with these, or when the patient is actually known to have subjected himself to the saturnine poison. Many of the symptoms are thus only corroborative of the rest, and if found isolated, would not deserve the same amount of attention.

It is easy to fill a book with cases, and, with very little trouble, an immense quantity of cases of lead colic and paralysis, emanating from the use of bad water, might be collected. Even from my own case-book, I could bring together more than the reader might care to peruse. Medical cases are highly valuable for reference, and they are always read with more interest when consulted in this way, than when read in the general perusal of a book. Instead of multiplying cases, however, I have sought only to set before the reader a selection which shall illustrate the different phases of the complaint, and I have purposely, in many instances, chosen the published cases of others, in preference to my own, that I may not appear either to want the support of others, or to forget the services they have rendered to mankind.

In September, 1848, I was requested to visit a servant girl who was suffering from violent pains in the bowels and from constipation. The pain was incessant. From the experience which I had previously had in the symptoms of lead colic, I imagined her disorder to be such. She vomited constantly, and tossed uneasily in bed, groaning with pain. There was not much tenderness of the abdomen, at least not more than the vomiting and griping would explain. To ascertain the state of the bowels in respect to tenderness, it is as well to make pressure gently and gradually, judging the effect rather from the countenance of the patient than by what is said. After the bowels had been well moved she became easier, and by taking small doses of Dover's powder, the pain was entirely removed. I explained to her the nature of the complaint, and she admitted having taken soft water from a lead cistern; but I did not examine the water. The pump belonging to the house was out of repair, and the water from it reputed to be bad. In March, 1849, I was asked to visit her again. She was in the same condition, in the same pain, with similar vomiting and constipation, but she seemed more wretched-looking, more sallow, and more emaciated. She had pain in the lower part of the back, and the gums were bordered with a deep blue line. I told her that she had not been attending to my directions, and with reluctance she confessed that such was the case. However, she seemed indisposed to attribute her complaint to the reputed cause, and looked somewhat dissatisfied with what I told her.

In July, 1849, she had another seizure. She had become sickly-looking, walked feebly, and was of a yellow complexion; there was the same colic and the same constipation. When I spoke of lead, she smiled with a look of incredulity. I was really provoked at her want of belief; but seeing the miserable condition to which she was reduced, I felt obliged to give her my professional aid. I took great pains to instruct her on the subject, and lent her some books, and a pamphlet which I had published, to inform her further as to the complaint. I also took occasion to speak to the lady, who was the housekeeper, (it being the house of a widower,) but I met with little support. It was stated that others took the same water without injury; and, in the end, only a sort of cold assent was given to my injunctions.—I shall, no doubt, surprise the reader with the continuance of my narrative, but I speak only the truth, which is sometimes more marvellous than fiction.—In March 27, 1850, she was ill again in the same way. She sent for me, being in great pain, and told me that she had done so with much reluctance; that she had been to consult another medical man since my last visit, who told her that her complaint originated in a diseased liver; and I scarcely wonder at his being deceived by the sallowness of her complexion. I told her that I would not prescribe for her any more, unless she attended better to my instructions, which she promised to keep. After a few months, in September, 1850, she had again a bad attack of lead colic, and, during my attendance at the house, another servant became affected in the same way,—the last person had not been long in the house, and indeed my former patient was the only servant who had been so. I think my patient was herself struck with the similarity of the complaint in her fellow servant. I was resolved, on this occasion, to investigate the matter fully, and then require implicit obedience, or refuse further attendance. I accordingly furnished myself with some water, charged with sulphuretted hydrogen gas, and took it to the house, with a view to test the water which the family were in the habit of using. I perceived some hesitation about the bringing of the water, and was eventually told that there was none of the drinking water in the house. I insisted on being shown what was usually taken, and the source from which it was taken. At length the servant said,—"I see, Sir, it's no further use deceiving you;" and then she took me into the scullery, and from a tap drew some hot water. She assured me that this was the only water used, and that it was suffered to cool for drinking;—that it was used regularly for tea, and that her master, a Greek gentleman, took it daily. On testing it, the water became of a dark brown colour, almost like coffee. I found it was conveyed from a lead cistern into the boiler behind the fire-place, and from this boiler, by a lead pipe, into the scullery. I believed this time that I had made some impression, but in order to guard still further against bad water, I directed her to live on a milk diet. Under this treatment she improved surprisingly, and recovered her usual looks; but she was unwilling to admit that it was owing to the disuse of the water. The family subsequently left the neighbourhood, but before she went she was well looking, and free from disease.

This case is perhaps as interesting from the obstinacy of the patient as from any other circumstance. Many times I doubted whether I had not mistaken the cause, for I could scarcely believe, after so many injunctions, and so painful an experience, that the patient would persist in the same course; but the trouble of fetching water, and a natural obstinacy of disposition, prevailed over all. This case may serve to show medical men how important it is, not to trust to the patient, where ignorance, prejudice, or indolence may operate. Some of this water I transmitted to the Board of Health, through the Honorable Mr. Napier, along with some MS., containing a notice of this and other cases; but the MS. was never used, and I have been unable to recover it after many endeavours.

In this case, too, it is important to observe that the two servants were the only patients; or if the gentleman was affected, he did not consult me, and his case was probably never understood. The children might have escaped, as they often do, by their milk diet. During my attendance on this case, my attention being drawn to the subject of lead, I discovered that another of my patients was suffering from the same cause. I shall briefly relate the case.

A gentleman who had been from home,

(January, 1849,) returned unexpectedly, suffering from ill health. On my arrival at the house he seemed a good deal agitated, and expressed a fear that he was going to have an inflammation of the chest. On the next day the pain had left the chest and seemed to be in the kidneys. On the third day he became more restless, complained of pains in his limbs, and was delirious. The skin perspired freely, and the bowels responded to medicine; there was a lateritious sediment in the urine. The delirium seemed aggravated by anodynes, which did not procure sleep. The illness continued many weeks, but in March he was sufficiently recovered to go to Bath, which he did by my advice. On his return from Bath he became somewhat worse, complained of rheumatic pains, and looked sallow. One day when he called upon me, I was struck with the half paralytic manner in which he dragged his legs up the steps at the front of the door. I then requested to examine the water he was in the habit of drinking, and I found it contaminated with lead. It was from a lead pump, and the family directed that it should be filtered for household use; but it is more than probable that it was not always filtered. This gentleman entered with great readiness into my views, and it was a pleasing exception to the indifference I have generally met with.

Whether the whole of his illness was dependent on the poison of lead, I will scarcely undertake to say, but the gentleman got well after he gave up the water; and it is certain that he suffered from the lead. Probably some of these less marked cases are the most instructive.

On Sunday, January 18th, 1852, I was requested to visit a gentleman who it was said had recently had a fit. The day previous, early in the morning, he had sent his carriage for me, but I had declined going, being engaged at the time, and thinking the distance too far conveniently to attend. His wife had died some time before, I think in December, (1851,) or thereabouts. I found him insensible. He was tossing from side to side. His hands were drawn and bent on the wrists, and the thumbs turned to the palms of the hands. Whilst feeling his pulse I perceived that there was a catching of the tendons. Any attempt made to look at the pupil of the eye caused him to draw away his head, and the same difficulty was experienced in any effort to examine the teeth, gums, or tongue. It was said that he had complained of pain in the stomach and bowels, but firm pressure seemed to cause no uneasiness, and was not resisted; nor was any impatience manifested on the examination. He rose up frequently into a sitting position, and made abortive efforts to vomit, then turned suddenly round in bed, and, after a short time, repeated this action. His complexion was of a yellow cast. His tongue, as far as I could see it, was clèan. His head was cool,—certainly not hot; all attempts to get any reply to questions were in vain. The pulse was not rapid,—there was no blue margin round the teeth. I suspected that he was suffering from lead, but having visited several pumps about the house, found that they were none of them objectionable, and the family denied having made use of the rain water. I still, however, suspected that the complaint was from lead. I got some croton oil, and gave two drops of it in a pill with crumb of bread; then I put four drops in some gruel, and administered it as an enema. I had difficulty in introducing the syringe from the contraction of the sphincter, and the injection did not seem to pass well, but came back again. At a subsequent period of the day I gave him two drops more of the croton oil in gruel, forcing the spoon between his teeth. After doing this, I went down stairs, but was soon called up again. I found that he was making an effort to get up, though quite unconscious; and thinking that he might be wishing to use the night chair, I desired that he might be assisted. When he got up he seemed very feeble, and not able to support himself without assistance. He did not part with any evacuation, and immediately tried to get into bed again, which he could not do without support. The man-servant, who was in the room assisting him, remarked that he rubbed his hand over his stomach. I turned down the clothes on several occasions, and verified his observation. Some few leeches were directed to be applied to the temples; but they were perhaps unnecessary. A dissenting clergyman who visited him, remarked, as he came down stairs, that he was very like, in complexion, to the lady, his wife, who had recently died. He continued the whole of the evening unconscious, but about 12 o'clock at night, the bowels acted, and he became slightly conscious.—He had been unconscious since early in the morning.

When I visited him the next day, I was shown a copious evacuation of a darkish colour. He was now partially conscious,—but he did not seem fairly to recognise me; yet, on being told to put out his tongue, he did so, and replied to questions after some little hesitation. I omitted to state that I applied a blister to the neck, and he first showed his consciousness by alluding to his neck when I asked him if he felt any pain. During this day, Monday, the bowels were plentifully acted upon. There was no vomiting, and no pain in the head.—He was not aware of what had transpired.—I gave him no medicine, with the exception of a spoonful of castor oil, and directed him to be kept on chicken, or mutton broth, or gruel, and farinaceous food.

As my visit was paid early in the morning, I found his sister, Miss —, taking her breakfast, and I noticed that a jug was on the table containing hot water for the supply of the tea-pot. I asked permission to examine this water, and poured some of it out into a tumbler to cool;—when it was cold I tested it with sulphuretted hydrogen gas water, which I had brought with me for the purpose, and I found that it showed indications of lead. I then asked for some of the pump water, which I likewise tested, but found it free from contamination. I then told the family that the water was evidently not from the spring, but was soft water; and, going into the kitchen, I found, by the side of the kitchen grate, a tap, which communicated with a boiler that always contained hot water. This I at once suspected to be the water which the family had used, and it was admitted by the servants to have been occasionally made use of to fill the kettle, and for other purposes. I took some of it home with me and tested it again, and found it very much contaminated.[1] It appeared, on inquiry, that the illness of the late Mrs. — had been attended with symptoms very similar to those of her husband, namely,— pains in the stomach, sickness, vomiting, and sallow complexion; and, finally, epileptic convulsions, and insensibility. Both Mr. and Mrs. — had been affected with a faltering in their speech, and Mr. — had been noticed to walk badly. Previous to his illness, Mr. — had eaten a hearty dinner with his brother, though at the time out of health.

[1] Subsequently the servant-man confessed to having used this water to fill the kettle.

On the third day, Wednesday, the 21st, Mr. — had no pains in the bowels nor head, but complained of aching pains in the limbs, not confined to the joints. His tongue was clean. He did not remember having sent for me, although, at the time he did so, he was perfectly conscious; so that previous events seemed abolished by his complaint. I understood that, for a long period before the attack, he had complained of shortness of breath, as well as of constant sickness and vomiting.

The day following he remained much as before. He was easy, with the exception of pains in his legs and arms, and said that he was feeble, and could not recollect what had passed. He seemed, as he had done previously, out of spirits, and inclined to remain quiet, as if asleep; but he was not asleep in reality, and said that his nights were not spent in repose, but that he only dozed and awoke at short intervals. I tested the water again in the presence of the domestics, and was myself surprised at the very decided change that was produced by the sulphuretted water. The bowels had been opened again since my last visit, but I recommended that purgatives should be continned, unless the bowels were naturally moved. I also still insisted on a very light, and, for the most part, farinaceous diet.

I was given to understand that a servant had recently left the house in a state of bad health, and had subsequently died, having, I believe, pains in her stomach and bowels; but it appears that she was of delicate and perhaps consumptive habits. Her friends, however, had expressed a belief, that there was a resemblance in her case to that of her mistress. I was further informed that the mother of Mrs. —, an elderly lady, who was accustomed to spend a month or more at a time with her daughter, had also lately died; but I cannot say how far the symptoms of her disorder coincided with those noticed in the other instances.

The servant-maid, who at present resides with the family, (Jan. 22, 1852,) seems in good health, and does not complain of any illness, with the exception of a pain at the lower part of the spine; but she has the blue discoloration at the borders of the gums in so marked a degree, that I think there can be little doubt that she suffers from lead contamination. In answer to some questions I asked her, respecting her fellow-servant, she told me that the young woman had complained of violent pains in the stomach and bowels, which rendered her unable to follow her work, and made her always restless in bed, and at times she "tossed about" in great pain. She seemed somewhat reluctant, however, to enter into particulars. With respect to the old lady, she could give me little information, and did not seem disposed to regard her case as similar; probably it was not so.—For her own part, she confessed that she had intolerable pain in the lower part of the spine.

Some time after the occurrence of these cases, I was in company with a lady who had resided in the same neighbourhood; she told me that she had been long an invalid, and was unable to procure any relief from her medical adviser; when hearing of the case which I have related, she made inquiries, and found that she was taking water from lead pipes. She discontinued its use, and got well. Another person was saved from a similar illness by the representations of one who had formerly been a patient of mine; so that the indirect good arising from these statements and cases, may, probably, be as great as is the immediate advantage to those concerned.

People who drink contaminated water from the kitchen boiler, must get their water mostly at their breakfast and tea; for at other times they are less likely to require it hot. Hence people often say that tea does not agree with them, and actually abandon it under this impression. Green tea, it is true, is often adulterated; but, I suspect, the water is more frequently to be blamed.

In March, 1852, I was requested by a lady to pay a professional visit to two of her servants, and she remarked that it was odd that *two* of them should be ill at the same time. One, a servant-lad, had obstinate vomiting and colicy pains. I noticed a dark reddish line round some of his teeth, and the interspaces were of a bluish cast. He complained of pain in the back, and great weakness of his legs, and said that he had several times been troubled with the same complaint. The other servant was the cook. She, likewise, was ill with pains in the bowels, but particularly in the lower part of the spine, and said that she was so weak that she could scarcely stand. When I conversed with her mistress below stairs, she asked me whether the cook was really so ill as she pretended to be; for, though she always complained of great weakness, she did not seem weak. Her gums bore striking evidences of the presence of lead. I thought this a good opportunity to question the cook as to whether she made use of the boiler-water; and I readily obtained an admission that she was in the habit of doing so. The servant-lad afterwards complained of pain in the shoulders,—told me that his legs were weak, and that, on moving or stooping, he still felt pain. The lady of the house had recently suffered from violent colicy pains, but they were attributed to food which she had taken; yet, it seems to me probable, that the food had disagreed simply because the bowels were partially paralysed.

In 1846 I attended a young gentleman for what I considered to be a rheumatic affection, and which yielded after a time. He then resumed his usual habits; but one day he was seized with a sudden pain in his bowels, and, as this did not pass off, I was again requested to attend. He had partaken the day before of some goose, to which the pain was attributed, particularly as he had eaten heartily of it. I ordered him some purgative medicine, but it only seemed to augment the pain. He did not appear to suffer much from direct pressure on the abdomen, but any motion of his body increased his uneasiness. After a time he got worse; a constant aching, griping pain, was complained of night and day. The bowels were not moved, though he took a great quantity of opening medicine. I now began to suspect that he had been drinking water contaminated with lead. I accordingly inquired whether the family made use of soft water for drinking, but was told that they did not. I further asked whether their pump was of lead, and being informed that this was not the case, I began to doubt the truth of my suspicion. However, the symptoms became more and more severe, so that I was led to repeat the question, and was then desired, in rather a dissatisfied manner, to examine the matter for myself. I found, after all, that the pump, which was placed in the cellar, was a leaden one, boxed round, as is usual, with wood; and further, that it was so far out of repair, that before water could be obtained from it, it was necessary to pour a considerable quantity of rain water into it by lifting off the top. The water used for this purpose was obtained immediately from a lead cistern. I now tested the water, and found it strongly impregnated with lead.

In the mean time, the young gentleman had become so far reduced in strength that I almost despaired of his life; he vomited every thing he took; the abdomen was tympanitic, and his limbs greatly emaciated; his pain was unceasing. During his illness he had complained much of thirst, and had taken copious draughts of the same water which had occasioned his disease. Having called in other medical men to confirm my views, and remove the surprise and doubts of the family as to the cause I assigned for the illness, the treatment was persevered in, and the young gentleman speedily recovered. I have seldom, in the course of my practice, seen a recovery effected under such unpromising appearances. In this case it was reasonably enough objected, in the first instance, that if lead were the cause of the disease, other members of the family would have suffered, who were also taking the same water.—This objection, however, need not detain us after what has been said.

Before I was properly aware of the symptoms of lead disease, I remember meeting with a case which I did not at first understand; having no notes of it, I must relate what I can from memory. I was requested to visit a young woman who was a servant in Broughton; she complained of pain in the back and bowels, vomited frequently, and was constipated. The pulse was quick, and the tongue clean, and I did not think she looked very ill or emaciated. I thought her representations were scarcely borne out by the symptoms, and her mistress hinted that she might be in a state of pregnancy. After a time, as she got no better, she was sent away, evidently under an impression that she had not been correct in her conduct. I was asked, however, to visit her at her own house, and the first time I did so, it struck me that her symptoms were produced by the poison of lead. The gums presented the blue line already mentioned, and there was, indeed, no doubt of the nature of the case; nor would there have been at the commencement, if I had been better acquainted with the subject. I thought it, therefore, my duty to call on the family with whom she had resided, in order to remove any unfavorable impression which might exist respecting the character of the servant. My representation was, however, received with evident distrust, and the lady of the house assured me somewhat coldly "that it was not her wish that the servants should drink soft water; and she conceived that she was as particular in these respects as her neighbours."

That the symptoms of lead colic, independently of chemical evidence, are almost sufficient in themselves to establish the existence of the poison, will appear from the following case:—A young woman, who was a servant in Broughton, was taken ill in August, 1850. She was feeble, somewhat emaciated, and, as she thought, bilious; she vomited all she took, and had pain at the lower part of the spine. The bowels were constipated. The medicine she took, was at first rejected by the stomach, but at length the disorder was overcome. I was struck at the time with the resemblance of the case to one of lead colic, but I could not trace the complaint to contaminated water. My own impression, however, was, that it arose from lead, and I was induced to entertain this idea from various other particulars, into which it is almost needless to enter. It afterwards appeared that this woman, who had not long been in her place, had lived at the house of a Greek gentleman, who I knew had a lead pump, the water from which was contaminated.

Whilst engaged in these inquiries concerning lead, a gentleman, who is an eminent engineer in Manchester, told me that his father, who was at an advanced age, had lost the use of his limbs. He described a kind of paralysis, which I thought it possible, might be of a saturnine origin; and without presuming that it was so, I desired him to write to his father, to inquire respecting the kind of water which he drank. In reply, it was stated that he drank soft water, and that the water was kept in a leaden cistern. He was advised to give up taking it, and in the end the paralysis disappeared.

This gentleman afterwards informed me that he had heard of three deaths arising from contaminated water. He stated that his informant was a reverend gentleman, who conducted the funeral services at a cemetery near Manchester. I went to the cemetery, and saw the clergyman, who told me that he had certainly interred *two* persons who were *said* to have died from such contamination, and he referred me to the medical gentleman who had attended them. I saw Mr. ——, the surgeon, who, with great candour and good sense, related to me the details of two cases, which were of so obscure a nature, that the true cause of the malady was not discovered until after death, though he was associated in the treatment with another medical man of considerable reputation. It was in the end found that the mischief proceeded from a lead pump, which, being pulled up, was found greatly corroded, and the water strongly impregnated with lead.

It would be well if every medical man had the same candour as the one to whom I allude. There were many circumstances which made it difficult for him to ascertain the real nature of these cases; and though he cannot be censured for not sooner arriving at the true nature of the complaint, he may surely be praised for his ingenuous relation. The brief memoranda with which he furnished me were unfortunately lost, with the MS. to which I alluded, as having been sent to the Board of Health, through the Honorable Mr. Napier.

Dr. Christison was kind enough to transmit me a paper, which he read before the Royal Society of Edinburgh, in February, 1842, and which is published in the Edinburgh Transactions: it contains an interesting case of lead colic which occurred to the housekeeper who resided at the cottage residence of the Earl of Aberdeen. The housekeeper was affected with indigestion and constipation, and was visited professionally by Mr. Johnston, of Peterhead, under whose directions she speedily recovered. Six weeks afterwards he was again sent for. She was troubled with vomiting, constipation, spasmodic pains, and great weakness of the limbs. He treated the case judiciously, but yet no permanent relief followed. At last, whilst considering the circumstances of his patient's illness, his attention was attracted by the incrustation which he saw on the water, in the water-bottle on the dressing-table. He was told that the water always presented this appearance after standing a short time, although it was transparent when first drawn. He had never seen a case of lead colic, but was at once struck with the possibility of this being such. He accordingly proceeded to make a chemical investigation, which led him to verify his suspicion. A niece of the housekeeper was also attacked with the premonitory symptoms, but recovered under Mr. Johnston's care. It appeared that the water was conducted to the house from a spring by a lead pipe, from a distance of rather more than half a mile, and had been in use for several months before the housekeeper went to reside at the lodge. But the water was of unusual purity, and continued all the while to receive impregnation. Dr. Christison states that the architect, under whose direction the water had been introduced, was slow to believe that the mischief really did arise from the lead; and he continues:—"It was plausibly argued that such accidents had not been observed in other places, and more especially at Aberdeen, where lead is prevalently used for conducting water."

To illustrate how easily this source of disease may escape the attention of the best informed, I am kindly permitted by Dr. Norris to relate some particulars of his own case; and it will, perhaps, be remembered that Dr. Norris has himself given much attention to the diseases produced by lead, and written ably on the subject. I shall make a short extract from his letter:—"If you think my own case sufficiently interesting, I will with pleasure give it you. * * * Some six or seven years ago I began to suffer with a dull griping pain in the bowels, and with symptoms of indigestion, though my digestion had formerly been remarkably good. These symptoms returned irregularly, but for the last few years were more continuous and severe. They seemed augmented by fatigue or anxiety, and were relieved by laudanum and weak brandy and water. The tongue was furred, and a rough sensation produced by the contact of the teeth, similar to that occasioned by acids. I had pain in the muscles, and particularly in the deltoid and large muscles of the lower extremities. My countenance had a sallow tinge. At one time I had a neuralgic pain in the forehead, and an amaurotic affection of the right eye. I found it necessary to lead a quiet, rather sedentary life, but daily followed professional avocations, avoiding, however, cases which required unusual exertion or anxiety. It is strange that I had been writing for several years on the more acute forms of lead disease, and never suspected the cause of my own suffering,—nor did my medical friends. After my last paper appeared in print, I accidentally discovered a leaden pipe hidden in a wall that conveyed water from the leaden pump of a neighbour into my own pump by an iron spouting. I immediately examined my gums, and found the blue tinge, which had doubtless been greater; for a month or so previously the pump had ceased to yield water, and I had already improved in health. Since the cause has been removed, my health has been re-established,—now for many months. If my symptoms did not arise from lead, from what can they have arisen?"[1]

Some most interesting examples of disorder produced by the poison of lead occurred at Claremont in 1848, in the distinguished French family who were resident there.[2] The cases are related in the 'Dublin

[1] Dr. Norris has since informed me that the water was examined and found to contain lead, and that he was, in some measure, led to the discovery by reading the author's pamphlet.

[2] The family and attendants of the late Count de Neuilly, ex-king of the French.

Quarterly Review' for 1849, by Dr. H. G. De Mussy. Dr. Mussy was summoned to Claremont in the beginning of October, 1848, and found one of the members of this family suffering from colic. He had a sallow complexion, a wasted condition of the body, and an anxious countenance. Within the last few weeks he had suffered frequent attacks of colic, nausea, and irregularity of the bowels. Dr. Mussy was somewhat uncertain about the nature of the illness, but was led to regard it as dependent on a derangement of the liver. Whilst attending his patient, a brother of the invalid became ill with the same symptoms; but this did not excite much attention, as it was supposed that he was suffering from a liver complaint contracted on the western coast of Africa. He had the same yellow cast of the conjunctivæ. A third patient, of 48 years of age, had suffered from colic a few days before, attended with nausea, vomiting, and obstinate constipation; but these had been attributed to a change of climate. Dr. Mussy remarks—"I must confess, even to my shame, that it did not occur to me to bring these three cases together, and to ascribe their similar symptoms to a single cause." A few days elapsed, and the patients were able to pursue their usual avocations, but were still feeble and had sallow complexions.

After about ten days, the patients again became ill with distressing pains in the bowels, constriction of the epigastrium, anxiety, nausea, and eructations. The constipation became more obstinate, the skin cold, and the pulse small and frequent. In one of the cases, (and Dr. Mussy remarks that it is worthy of notice, as being unusual,) the sphincter vesicæ did not admit the urine to pass off for more than thirty-six hours, so that the bladder extended up to the umbilicus, and excruciating pains were experienced in the back and loins, &c. But the nervous symptoms were the most frightful to witness—the patients were restless in bed and unable to find an easy position—hysteric symptoms came on, and the patients shed tears and uttered groans, less from the violence of their pains than from their uncontrollable feelings. Excessive sensibility of the body also arose, so acute, that the slightest touch gave extreme pain, and extorted cries from the sufferers. This sensibility frequently changed its position, and seemed to appear and re-appear in a capricious manner. It existed chiefly on the surface of the body, and was more excited by a slight touch than by a firm pressure; though it was evidently most apparent over the osseous projections of the spine:—this circumstance probably arose from the skin being at these parts more amenable to pressure. In two other patients, who afterwards became affected, this sensibility was almost the only symptom noticed.—One was a female of nervous and lymphatic constitution, whose constipation was readily relieved, but whose excessive sensibility continued three days. The other, a young man of twenty-four, never experienced either colic or constipation, but complained, during several days, of excessive pain in the parietes of the thorax, greatly increased by a slight touch, or even by the respiratory movements. In the same patient the hysteric symptoms were also strongly marked, and he gave way to sighs, groans, and abundant tears. Dr. Mussy says—"Certainly, if these symptoms had been present in *this case only*, unaccompanied by any other phenomena of more importance, I never should have attributed them to the disease to which they truly belong." Dr Mussy now examined the gums of his patients, and found the blue line which has been mentioned, and, in some, slate-coloured spots in the inside of the mouth. Dr. Rieken, physician to the King of the Belgians, having arrived at Claremont, also visited the patients, and concurred with Dr. Mussy in concluding that the diseases arose from the poison of lead. They accordingly proceeded to test the water with a solution of sulphuretted hydrogen; but either owing to the test not being good, or what is more likely, to their not being furnished with the water really taken, no precipitate was found. Sir James Clark, calling the next day, to inquire after the inhabitants of Claremont, kindly undertook to send specimens of the water to Professor Hoffman, who immediately detected a considerable quantity of lead in it, so that the pipes which brought the water to the palace were immediately cut off. In the mean time the patients continued to suffer, notwithstanding active and judicious treatment. Dr. Mussy gave small doses of ice, and croton oil in pills, as much as eight minims of the latter in twenty-four hours. This produced dark and copious evacuations, but relief did not invariably follow. The patients became greatly emaciated and cachetic looking, and were troubled with abundant sweats. One patient had several convulsions; and in another, the sight became so weak that Dr. Mussy feared amaurosis. Dr. Mussy thought at this period that it was desirable to abandon the drastic purgatives, and resort to belladonna and opium, repeated every four or six hours, with small pieces of ice; and afterwards a weak infusion of rhubarb. Fresh patients now began to suffer, but less severely than those already affected. Those first attacked, remained still cachetic, emaciated, and in some degree paralytic. Sulphurous baths were prescribed every second day, and the chemical action shewed itself by the blackening of the nails of the feet and hands, and some parts of the skin. The presence of lead was even detected in the urine. Dr. Mussy could not fail to observe, that the poison did not act on all the patients with the same degree of intensity; but he was not surprised at this, as he knew that some workmen are able to resist the influence of lead for many years, and others are affected from the very beginning.

Few instances could be found which exemplify more clearly the effects of lead in its different forms: there were thirty-eight inhabitants at Claremont, and of these, thirteen were attacked, eleven men and two women. Four were ill two months before Dr. Mussy's arrival, and the other cases occurred under his eyes. Some were affected even after the supply of water was cut off, and one, a week after leaving England. Six children, aged from three to seven, were exempt.

Only one half the patients had the slate-coloured mark on the gums; and others, who did not experience any inconvenience from the lead, had indications of it in the condition of the gums. The malady, as will be easily supposed, shewed "no respect for condition, and attacked indiscriminately servants, aides-de-camp, and princes, and did not spare even the most august and pious of victims."

The spring which furnished the palace at Claremont, issued from a sand-bed about two miles distant. It was chosen for its great purity about thirty years ago, and was conducted through lead pipes. The inhabitants had used it for many years without bad effects, and it was not a little singular that it should afterwards have become injurious. It seems, however, that some recent alterations had been made, which might, perhaps, account for this effect. Since the present occupants of the palace had arrived, the natural cistern which received the water, had been furnished with an iron cylinder, in order to preserve it from the vegetable matter, which usually fell into it, and, it is possible, that something was attributable to a galvanic action, resulting from the contact of the metals with the water.

In the 'Edinburgh Monthly Journal of Science,' for May, 1852, there is an interesting paper by Dr. George Wilson, on the poisoning of horses by lead. He commences his paper in these words;—"The destruction of animal life, which yearly results from the mismanagement of chemical works in rural places, is probably greater than is generally imagined. Within the short space of five months, last year, I had occasion to make a series of analyses in connection with the death of thirteen horses, which, besides several cows, were believed to have been poisoned by compounds of lead transferred by the atmosphere, or by water, to the fields in which they pastured. How far the conclusion was just," continues the writer, "which imputed the death of all these animals to lead-poisoning, I cannot pretend to decide, as analyses were made in connection only with some of the cases; but as I found the herbage which the animals ate, was notably impregnated with carbonate of lead, it is highly probable that all the deaths were occasioned by this poison." In conclusion, Dr. Wilson remarks, 1st,—that as all the organs of the body of the horses which he examined contained lead, it appears to him, that lead, in cases of slow poisoning, exerts its influence generally, though it may be unequally, on the different parts; and, 2dly, that when lead has once entered the body, it leaves it again very slowly, and long after the system has ceased to receive the contaminated food or drink.

On one occasion, when I was attending a servant-girl for an attack of lead colic, produced by contaminated water, the master of the house inquired, whether it was possible for horses to be injured by drinking the same. I told him that I saw no reason why they should not be affected with it; and he then told me, that ever since he had resided at his present house, the horses were restless and given to kicking in the stable, in a manner that he could not account for. As many people are more careful of their horses than themselves, the hint may not be lost.

It is of particular importance to remark, that it is not sufficient to content ourselves with inquiries concerning the source of the water taken, nor always, indeed, with the inspection of the well or pump supposed to be used. We may be allowed to entertain doubts whether water may not be occasionally taken, which is derived from other places. In illustration of these remarks, I may allude to a valuable communication made to the Lancet, by Dr. James Robertson, physician to the Hitchin Infirmary.

At a school, where about twenty girls were educated, and where every attention was scrupulously paid to health and regularity, it was observed that many of the scholars fell into a state of disease. The rest of the inmates, who seemed to be placed in precisely similar circumstances, remained well; so that Dr. Robertson was unable to account for this disorder. The girls lost their healthy colour, and became pale; their appetites failed, and their breath became offensive. Some had occasional diarrhœa, and some obstinate constipation. For several months the general health declined, though no cause was apparent.—The diet was changed and improved, and medicine was taken, but without relief. One girl was, at times, delirious, and several had fits, described as hysterical. These illnesses caused Dr. Robertson to examine, again and again, carefully, the food and water, but he was unable to find anything in them deleterious.

At length, Dr. Robertson's attention was attracted to a lead cistern which supplied water for the girls' washing-place, though he was assured that this water was never used except for washing. Thinking, however, that it was conveniently situated for the play-ground, he imagined that it might be used contrary to orders. This, in fact, proved to be the case, and it was àt length admitted by the girls, that they were in the constant habit of drinking it, when no fresh water was at hand. The water was found to contain an abundance of lead; even that which was filtered, contained a small quantity, though so small, that, at the first examination, it escaped detection. After the children ceased to drink the water, they rapidly improved — the amendment being decidedly evident even three weeks after the discovery.[1]

I know it will be allowed that there is

[1] Dublin Medical Press, vol. xxv, p. 153.

much truth in what I have written,—but, I fear, it may be supposed that there is also some exaggeration. Let it be remembered, however, that the appearance of exaggeration may depend on a real ignorance, on the part of the objectors, to the extent of the mischief, of which I speak. It was many years before I had myself arrived at a full comprehension of the importance of this subject; and let not the conviction, which has sprung from eight or ten years careful and cautious investigation, be pronounced unfounded without a similarly long and cautious inquiry. I may possibly incur the ridicule of superficial thinkers, but I do not fear to incur that of the true and patient observers of disease. Perhaps some may be deterred from the study of lead affections, because the subject may seem to be a peculiarly dry one; but, it will be found in reality to be one of especial interest, because the cases of lead disease are, more than all others, striking in their results. In some instances acute colic is speedily cured; but what is still more remarkable, a steady and chronic ailment shall be eventually removed; a painful disease, a slow wasting of the body, or dragging palsy, shall be finally dispersed. I feel particular confidence in speaking of the importance of the subject, because I am certain that these effects are within the compass of treatment, and that a very large class of apparently anomalous cases owe their origin to the poison of lead. If there be reluctance, on the part of the profession, or of the public, to credit these statements, it is only the better proof how much they were needed; and, it must be remembered, that the labours of the distinguished Sir George Baker, were themselves only met with incredulity and distrust.

It is amusing to notice the absurd ingenuity with which writers, previous to the able researches of Sir George Baker, endeavoured to refer the colic of Poitou to any but the right source, and the reluctance with which they adopted the true pathology. Sir George Baker thus concludes an able paper, in which he comments on these points with his characteristic modesty,—a modesty which is most generally found where it is the least needed.—"I do not," says he, "affirm that there does not exist another cause productive of similar effects; but, from what has above been written, it may, perhaps, appear that such a supposition, (the colic of Devonshire, depending on the poison of lead,) is not void of probability; since no other cause has hitherto been shown to be adequate to the phenomena."[1]

Before I take leave of this part of the subject, I shall go back, once more, to some points, which I have wished, especially, to impress on the reader. It must be remem-

[1] Med.-Chir. Trans., vol. i, p. 406.

bered, in all cases where symptoms exist, which lead to the supposition of saturnine poisoning, that care be taken to look minutely for all possible sources of such contamination; and to bear in mind that these sources may, even, be in themselves of only occasional operation.

Examples of obscure disorder, so arising, will be strikingly seen, by attention to the diseases of domestics. There are many domestic servants who complain of constipation, debility, pain in the spine, and occasional colic. Their gums will be found bluish, and their complexions sallow. These patients are mostly in the habit of using the hot water from the kitchen boiler, but they do so, only when it is a matter of convenience. There is obstinate pain, sometimes, at the epigastrium, which does not yield to the usual remedies which are prescribed for gastrodynia. They imagine that the water is only objectionable from its not being quite so clean as the spring water; and they perhaps forget that it comes from the cistern, or do not know that such water would be injurious.

They use it for cooking, occasionally, and at least, boil the potatoes or the pudding in it. I have often asked servants about these matters, and by a little management have generally been candidly informed by them. It must be remembered that they act from ignorance; for they are generally themselves the chief sufferers;—at all events, the blame is not so great as it may appear, for, if the water did not receive contamination from lead, the other considerations would be comparative trifles. I have seldom found, that where a boiler containing hot water was easily accessible in the kitchen, it was not used for culinary purposes. I have generally had it easily admitted, but the admission must be gained by address. It is not well to find fault, as it immediately leads to denials, and closes the inquiry. We should state, in a friendly manner, that it has been found that water from a lead cistern produces great mischief, and add something of the symptoms which it occasions. We may then ask them to say, honestly, and without any fear of censure, whether they have not occasionally used it. If it be admitted that it has been used *occasionally*, we may feel tolerably sure that it has been *often* used.—I have thought it necessary to be thus particular, for I know it to be a very important matter to arrive at the real truth in these *apparently* frivolous matters.

Not seldom, two or three servants are taken ill at the same time, or consecutively; and the symptoms, in these cases, will be found to resemble each other, in many important points. It is true, there will be differences which would lead an inattentive observer to regard them as different complaints; but there will yet be left a striking similarity in many of the features. One person may be affected with colic, and be tolerably robust, and be only recently taken ill; another may be of a sallow complexion, and of an emaciated form, and may have been long complaining of indigestion, and of constipation; a third may have blue gums, uneasiness in the stomach, and be troubled with vomiting. The master and mistress of the house may be quite well, and the children perfectly so. Servants, for many reasons, are most likely to suffer. Many of them make tea or coffee, in small quantities, when the kettle has already been exhausted, using the boiler-water to replenish it. Many, from peculiar fancies, or from some perversion of appetite, make their meals of tea in preference to meat; some, from a similar reason, prefer the taste of the soft water. The master and the mistress may drink wine or malt liquor with their meals, and the children have milk. Servants will also be found differently affected, according to the length of time they have resided in the house:—some may have been one year,—others three or four. Those who have been the longest suffer the most in their general health, and look more emaciated, and feel more weak. It is often a matter of wonder that any one should suffer, where all appear to be placed in similar circumstances; but if *every circumstance* were known, how different would be the degrees in which the inhabitants of the same house have been exposed to the danger!

Independently of the contamination of water with the poison of lead, there can be no doubt but there are numerous other sources from which it may be derived; and I have myself a strong conviction that much disease, which is never properly understood, arises from the adulteration of food with lead. In the present age of refinement and luxury, this is an evil which it is almost impossible to avoid, though much might be done that has yet never been attempted.

"From a careful perusal," says Dr. Burton, "of the authors before named, (alluding to the papers of Sir George Baker and Dr. Warren,) as well as from considerable personal experience, I presume to express a strong belief that the unobserved introduction of lead into the human body is continually taking place to a much greater extent than is usually imagined, and that it has often caused an ambiguous assemblage of morbid symptoms; for although the influence of lead on the system is readily detected, when the symptoms are severe and follow each other in the expected order of succession, yet, when they are mild, or do not follow each other in the regular stated order of succession, if the mind of the physician is not awake to their cause, or the cause cannot be ascertained, then the symptoms appear ambiguous, and they may be misinterpreted without exposing the physician to the imputation of unpardonable ignorance, or of culpable oversight."[1]

Sir George Baker also had a similar suspicion, that deleterious effects might arise in a very insidious manner from the employment of lead. "Particularly is it not probable," says he, "that the bowels of children may frequently suffer from their food, in this manner impregnated with lead? And in general may it not justly be concluded, that some of the slighter disorders of the first passages may be the effects of a concealed poison? And may not some part of that benefit, which our health usually receives, on our quitting, for some time, the accustomed places of our residence, arise from the circumstance of our quitting the daily use of something deleterious, which we have

[1] Med.-Chir. Trans., vol. v, 2d series, p. 73.

been accustomed to swallow with our daily nourishment?"[1]

That Lead may be used safely as a medicine there can be no doubt, and, in many instances, it is found a most serviceable one. —In some cases of dysentery or protracted diarrhœa, it is of special utility. It seems, indeed, to be less injurious, when given for a short time in efficient doses, than when it is introduced in small quantities for a long period of time. When Lead is administered as a medicine, its effects are generally carefully watched by the practitioner, and the symptoms of colic, when they occur, are mostly met with promptitude, and easily removed. Dr. Radclyffe Hall, of Torquay, writes me word,—"In a case of severe hæmoptysis, where I gave ninety-six grains of *Plumbi Diacet.* in three days—thirty-two in the first four hours, the only unpleasant effect was a moderate pain in the bowels."

[1] Med.-Chir. Trans., vol. i, p. 277.

This, Dr. Hall was scarcely disposed to regard as the effect of the lead, though it probably was so in reality. It is always well, however, to bear in mind, in using lead internally, the possibility of its producing poisonous effects; and there can be no doubt, from what we read of the history of diseases in former times, that it was frequently fatal when employed as a curative agent.

It was, indeed, the doctrine of Paracelsus that "Saturnus purgat febres"—and we cannot then wonder, that colic and palsy were frequent results of fevers treated by preparations of lead.

A case is related from Carolus Piso, of a young man, who, from a tertian fever, fell into a quotidian, which endured forty days, and was then succeeded by a palsy in the arm, and afterwards by convulsions and death. But Carolus Piso mentions the termination of colic in palsy, as a common occurrence; and alluding to an observation made by his father, Nicholas Piso, mentions that in the province of Lorraine such a species of colic was particularly common, so that "it would be tedious to enumerate singly all the patients whom he had seen thus affected." Either from the administration of medicines, or the adulteration of wine, or water, the monks appear to have suffered much from saturnine poisoning. The same author, Carolus Piso, relates that he visited two convents; one in the year 1596, and the other seven years later. In both houses he found the monks most miserably affected; some with colic, others with palsied arms, which hung useless from the shoulders; others harassed with convulsions, and some in a comatose state. These effects, the author, from a preconceived theory, attributed to fever; but even *he* was obliged to confess that *the fever was valde mediocris.*

In the 'Dublin Medical Press' for January

14, 1852, a case is published from an American journal, as a caution respecting the medicinal use of the acetate of lead. Thirty grains of the acetate of lead were prescribed by Dr. Joynes, of Accomack, U. S., in about four days, for an inveterate diarrhœa. The medicine seemed to be of service, and the physician and his patient were congratulating themselves on the result, when, about a week after the discontinuance of the medicine, the patient was seized with pain in the epigastrium, and some time after, an attack of lead colic came on, and continued with more than ordinary severity for eight days. Calomel and opium were freely given until the mercury affected the mouth; which was probably carrying the remedy to an unnecessary extent.

Dr. Joynes, in commenting upon this case, remarks, that the opinion of Dr. A. T. Thomson, that the carbonate of lead is the only poisonous preparation, is opposed to the truth, and has been productive of much mischief in giving the profession an undue confidence in the protection afforded by acetic acid. It seems to me more in accordance with generally admitted views, to believe that the energy of a poison is in proportion to its solubility; and, as Dr. Joynes observes, before the carbonate can be prejudicial, it is most likely that it is converted into an acetate, or other soluble salt, by the action of the gastric juice.

I now come to speak of the treatment of the affections of lead, and I am glad to say that it is generally highly satisfactory. There is an adage, that a knowledge of a disease is half its cure; and certainly, a knowledge of the nature of a malady which arises from lead, is more than half contributive to the restoration of the patient.

In the treatment of lead affections we are obviously guided by the form and degree of the disorder; so that the subject naturally divides itself into the treatment of the various phases we have noticed, such as the saturnine colic, paralysis, and arthralgia.

In the treatment of lead colic, it is easy to suppose that the obstinate constipation, which attends the complaint, would readily suggest the employment of powerful purgatives,—whilst a wish to dislodge the poison from the system would give occasion to the use of emetics. Accordingly, we find the earlier writers on the subject, such as Celsus, Paulus Ægineta, and others, recommending the administration of emetics and purgatives. Subsequently, a similar mode of treatment became famous at the Hospital of La Charité; and even to the present day, this method has been handed down with various modifications, and has called forth the commentaries of all writers on the subject of lead.

Brachet says, after speaking of the early adoption of this plan,—" En 1602 ce traitement sembla prendre plus de régularité entre les mains des religieux italiens que Marie de Médicis avait fait venir pour gouverner l'hôpital de La Charité. Sous le nom de *macaroni*, ils employèrent un remède composé d'une partie de verre d'antimoine et de deux parties de sucre, le tout pulvérisé et bien mêlé: on le donnait à la dose d'un scrupule, trois ou quatre jours de suite. Les succès de ce remède contre la colique des peintres firent affluer à La Charité les malades qui en étaient atteints."[1] The medical men who succeeded these religious characters in taking care of the patients, continued the same line of treatment, with, however, such occasional modifications as experience seemed to point out. There can be little doubt, but that the system of proceeding, so celebrated at La Charité, was effective and useful; but, on the other hand, it is to be regretted that it was often

[1] Traité pratique de la Colique de Plomb, p. 164.

unnecessarily severe. In particular, perhaps, the use of emetics was uncalled for. Instead of accepting any method of treatment as a whole, it is proper to inquire into the nature of its elements, and seek to discover what may be omitted with advantage, and to what the efficacy of the prescription is principally owing.—Those who are anxious to read particulars of the famous treatment of La Charité, will find much on the subject in the works of Mérat, Tanquerel Desplanches, and M. Brachet.

Of the purgatives most efficient in lead colic, I think there can be little question that the croton oil (Croton Tiglium) takes the first place; and the readiness with which it can be given, notwithstanding the patient may be affected with obstinate vomiting, or even insensibility, is not a small recommendation in its favour. It is true many minor derangements from the poison of lead, will readily yield to the more lenient purgatives, such as castor oil, or the sulphate of magnesia; but the croton oil is by far the most efficient, where the constipatiou is obstinate. The employment of mercury as a purgative, does not seem essential; and certainly to give it with a view to salivation is as unnecessary as it is mischievous. The dose of the croton oil must vary with the exigencies of the case, and may be repeated, if not speedily successful. From one, to two, or three drops, may be administered at once, either with crum of bread, extract of colocynth, or any other convenient vehicle. It may be used also by injection with gruel, in doses of four or five drops. Where the croton oil is not effective, it may be necessary to suspend the purgative plan, and seek to relieve pain by the administration of opiates. The full evacuation of the bowels seems essential, however, before the cessation of the colic can be relied on. When the bowels have been evacuated, it is not to be supposed that everything is accomplished. The relief may be but temporary, and it is only by a continued attention to the evacuation of the bowels that the cure can be achieved. The paralysed state of the alimentary canal yet remains; and though the load it was unable to void may, in some degree, be removed, a part may yet remain, or future fæcal collections may soon be produced. Small doses of croton oil made into pills, with aloes or colocynth, should be taken once or twice in the day, for several days, if the bowels are not fully cleared without them; and the practitioner will do well, for some days, to inspect the evacuations for himself. I have found this necessary in the colic which proceeds from contaminated water.

Brachet, in his recent volume on Lead Colic, seems to think most highly of alum, which he believes to fulfil the *citò, tutò et jucundè,* of Celsus, more than any other remedy. He does not consider its beneficial effects to arise from its influence as a mere chemical agent. Nor does he wish to underrate the value of the purgative treatment, which he admits, but he imagines the alum to be less annoying to the patient, more safe, and more speedy in its operation. But he unites it with opiates, and follows its exhibition with purgatives. As I have not such opportunities of comparing the action of remedies as are afforded by the large French hospitals, I can only say that, in the colic produced by contaminated water, the purgative plan has appeared to me both safe and effective.

The great pain which accompanies the saturnine colic, has induced some practitioners to insist much on the advantage of anodyne remedies. Stoll, in particular, advocated them. He was led to rely upon this method of treatment from no preconceived theory, but from a case which occurred to him. He had been vainly endeavouring to relieve a patient, for many days, who vomited incessantly, and had no alvine discharge, at the same time that he was tortured with the most violent pains. Stoll was averse to the employment of opiates on account of the constipation they are known to produce; at length he was constrained, by the severity of the suffering, to resort to opiates, and the bowels were then relaxed, whilst the vomiting subsided. After this time he was encouraged to pursue the anodyne method, and, as he represents, with the best effects. That good may arise from opiates, there can be little doubt; there are few cases, however, that could be advantageously treated by them alone. Where opiates are indicated by the great violence of the suffering, unrelieved by active purgatives, or remaining after the evacuation of the bowels, considerable doses of opium may be given with advantage; and it is remarked by Tanquerel, that narcotism is not easily produced in the cases where they are necessary. Besides opium, other anodynes have, of course, been recommended, but many of them are, no doubt, less safe, such as belladonna, and tobacco. In estimating the effects of some of these, writers have not always borne in mind that the remedies were associated with others, or given when the cure was already in progress.

It can scarcely be supposed that in so painful a complaint as lead colic, bloodletting should have been neglected. Accordingly, we find numerous writers advocating its employment, amongst which were many of the disciples of Broussais. M. Tanquerel, who is never content to speculate on matters which can only be properly decided by a careful and philosophical experience, gives us the results of the antiphlogistic method in numerous cases which came under his observation. Of 84 patients who had been submitted to this treatment before their admission to La Charité, 60 suffered more at their entry than previously to treatment, 6 were relieved, and 18 remained in the same condition. "Le traitement antiphlogistique ne semble donc pas avoir une influence bien marquée sur le cours de la colique."

As the lead colic is not an inflammatory complaint, and is not accompanied in general with any tenderness of the abdomen, there seems no sufficient reason for the employment of bloodletting. It is possible that complications may sometimes render it necessary; but to pursue the antiphlogistic system, as a chief means of removing the disorder, does not seem consistent, either with enlightened experience or with sound pathology.

Chemical remedies for the disorders produced by lead, have naturally had many advocates, but it is a little singular that the advocacy has been maintained on exactly opposite views. Some have recommended agents, which, they imagined, would render the lead more soluble, and thus favour its elimination from the body; others have endeavoured to form insoluble salts of lead, and thus neutralise its deleterious influence. Certain bodies, which may be supposed to operate chemically, have been found useful; but experience, rather than theory, must decide upon their merits. The use of dilute sulphuric acid drinks, as a preventive of lead colic, and the employment of the sulphur bath, in the treatment of some forms of lead disease, may be instanced as valuable chemical means. Writers, of a physiological bias of mind, have regarded, what they conceived to be, the paralysed condition of the bowels as a principal consideration in the treatment of lead colic; and hence blisters, electricity, and the nux vomica have been resorted to. The utility of the latter in the *palsy* of lead has probably suggested its use in the *colic*. M. Tanquerel has given trial to this as well as other remedies, but does not decide favorably as to its use. Fourteen patients were submitted to this treatment; thirty drops of the alcoholic tincture were given them daily, *en lavement*, in decoction of marsh mallows. In the case of four who had the colic violently, no proper relief was gained after many days, and recourse was finally had to the croton oil. In the case of five who had it less severely, the amendment was slow, and some required the croton oil to complete the cure. Of the five others, only slightly affected, the treatment lasted six days, and one had a relapse, which required other means. These facts, says M. Tanquerel, speak sufficiently for themselves, and need no comments to prove that the nux vomica has no influence, or at least, only a slight one, on the course of lead colic, and that this medicine does not produce in this disease any purgative effect.

How far chloroform may be useful in the treatment of lead colic, it is perhaps, at present, premature to decide; but several fatal cases, which have occurred on the Continent, should serve as a caution to those who are inclined to employ it. Whilst the croton oil is found so safe and efficient, it is well to proceed with care in our inquiries into the utility of dangerous or uncertain means. From what has been said, then, it will appear, that, though good may arise in particular instances from various remedies, the use of efficient purgatives, and especially of the croton oil, furnishes the best means of relief; at the same time, pain may be assuaged, when necessary, by stupes, and warm fomentations to the abdomen; and the internal administration of opiates, in the intervals of rest.

To a certain extent, the same remedial means, which are necessary for the colic of lead, are desirable in the treatment of the other forms of lead disease which arise from contaminated water; and, for the most part, with the avoidance of the *cause*, and the regulation of the bowels, the cure is ultimately worked out. There are some affections which, however, in the mean time, demand attention, and some which would not readily yield without especial consideration. The *arthralgia* and painful contractions, which so frequently accompany lead disease, may themselves be exceedingly obstinate, and for these, the sulphur baths will probably be found the most serviceable. Tanquerel says,—"Pour obtenir les résultats les plus avantageux de l'administration des bains sulfureux, il faut les prescrire tous les jours, pendant sept à huit jours. Cinq à six onces de sulfure de potasse est la quantité de substance médicamenteuse mise dans chaque bain à La Charité."[1]

[1] Vol. i, p. 523.

Still more important, however, is the paralysis which results from lead, and still more urgently, therefore, may we be called upon to give it an individual treatment. It is to be hoped that a gradual improvement will be found to arise, where daily attention is given to the condition of the bowels, to the cleanliness of the skin, to exercise and diet, and the careful avoidance of the original cause; but, to render recovery more rapid, aid has been properly sought in various means. Stimulating embrocations have been recommended by some, and electricity and galvanism praised by others. The sulphurous baths have also been considered serviceable, but the medicine, which has acquired the greatest celebrity, is the vegetable alkali Strychnine, which was discovered by MM. Pelletier and Caventou. This medicine has the advantage of being easily administered, from the smallness of the quantity required, and may either be given in pills, or in a spirituous preparation. It must be remembered, however, that this medicine is an active poison; and I have always, myself, felt some degree of reluctance in having recourse to means which are dangerous in themselves. Strychnine should be given, at first, in small doses, and its effects carefully watched, and the preparation increased by degrees. If twitching is produced, it may be necessary to diminish the dose, or even to withdraw the remedy. The dose commonly prescribed is from one-tenth to one-eighth of a grain, and the effects are said to manifest themselves in two or three hours after it is taken.

I must confess that I should be afraid of pushing this medicine to the extent which some have recommended, and yet it is, no doubt, better tolerated in saturnine paralysis than in other diseases. But it is well to have constantly in mind, that the medicine may produce its effects suddenly, and with great activity; so that it is necessary to give a careful and continued attention to every patient who is submitted to its administration.

Where the body has already undergone an obvious atrophy of the muscular structure, it is almost unnecessary to say that less benefit is to be expected.

The cure of paralysis requires a much longer time than that of the colic, and one or two months may be regarded as an average period. In addition to other means, the muscular contractions may, in some measure, be obviated by mechanical contrivances. Dr. Pemberton proposed the use of splints, to prevent the undue influence of the flexor muscles; but how far they are really useful, I am unable to say.

If the practitioner do not wish to have recourse to strychnine, the nux vomica may be used, in combination with aloes; and Dr. Copland recommends this method in preference to the other. In amaurotic affections, the restoration of sight may, probably, be expedited by the application of blisters to the temples.

In epilepsy and coma, resulting from lead, the treatment must be allowed to be, in a great measure, of the *expectant* nature, at least after the evacuation of the bowels, and the adoption of the remedies which have been pointed out as most efficient in the colic. Active bleeding is not called for, and would even be positively injurious; but the application of blisters and sinapisms may be tried, with some prospect of advantage. Enemata may also be used with turpentine, or croton oil, particularly if it be thought that the bowels have not been sufficiently relieved.—It must be remembered that the coma is not one of simple congestion, and is not to be dealt with as an apoplectic seizure.

The treatment of the more *chronic* affections

produced by lead, must obviously embrace dietetic considerations, as well as the administration of medicine. The avoidance of all possible sources of saturnine contamination must be rigorously regarded; for quantities of lead which would scarcely, perhaps, be deleterious to the healthy, may be highly prejudicial to those already ill. But it is not sufficient to avoid these sources—it is necessary also to abstain from all common causes of indigestion, and from all articles of food and drink capable of producing any derangement. The stomach and bowels must be considered as paralysed in their functions, and incapable of fulfilling their natural actions. It is well to impress this repeatedly on the patient, for it is only by degrees that he can return, with safety, to his usual habits of living. It is also prudent to abstain from many things which may have possible adulterations with lead—for it would not be easy, in all cases, to enter upon a chemical examination of the different articles of food which are taken. On this account, I have thought it especially necessary to avoid wines, particularly what are called "made wines," or wines bought from dealers in small quantities. Without going so far as to say that all these wines may be suspected of adulteration, I would, at least, say that they are injurious to those who are only recently convalescent. A milk diet seems to me especially free from objection, and a steady continuance of such a regimen is generally attended with the greatest good.—A complaint which has been slow in its progress of development, may naturally be supposed to require time for its perfect removal; and, as a latent period seemed to exist before the manifestation of the disorder, so a latent period may be conceived to premise the perfect dissolution of the malady when formed.

As a watering place for the resort of convalescents, Bath has long enjoyed a reputation. Dr. Andrew informed Sir George Baker, that patients brought to the Devon and Exeter Hospital, who did not easily recover, were sent to the Bath Hospital. "I have known this complaint (says he, speaking of lead disease,) cured radically, though I confess a return often happens. —When the disease proves obstinate, we always endeavour to get our patients into the hospital at Bath; the Bath-water, though not a specific, being esteemed by us the most effectual remedy, both internally and and externally used."[1]

There are many other ways in which lead may be taken into the system, besides the drinking of contaminated water. These do not, properly, fall within the scope of my observations; but I should perhaps do wrong to omit a brief allusion to them, by way of appendix to what has been said. I shall, however,

[1] Med.-Chir. Trans., vol. i, p. 201.

make mention only of those which are met with in domestic life; for a consideration of the injurious effects of lead in the Manufactures, is, in itself, a comprehensive subject.

I may, perhaps, be permitted to repeat some of the observations which I have already offered on the subject, in a small tract which I published in 1850.

Wine bottles are often cleaned with shot, and it must sometimes happen that the shot itself will be left sticking to the inside of the bottle. A case is mentioned in the 'Lancet,' for the 20th of April, 1844, and is copied from the 'Journal de Chemie.' A person, who had drunk a few small glasses of liqueur, was seized with violent colic; Dr. Hanle, who was immediately called in, examined the remainder of the liquid, which was found of a dirty hue. Some lead shots were discovered fixed at the bottom of the bottle, and almost corroded.

Sometimes, however, lead is purposely

used in the manufacture of home-made wines. Sir George Baker actually mentions a receipt "to *hinder wine from turning*," which directs a pound of melted lead to be put in the cask. It is given under the article of "Secrets belonging to the Mystery of Vintners," in a book written by one William Graham, as a sort of small compendium of housewifery.[1]

It is well known that milk is not unfrequently kept in leaden troughs, in order that the cream may be collected. Dr. Darwin relates the case of a young woman who was seized with colic and paralysis, and eventually died from "*licking*" the cream so collected;—she was a farmer's daughter. On this case, Dr. Christison remarks, that lead appears sometimes to be used, for the purpose named, with safety, but will, of course, be dissolved, if the milk become sour."[2]

[1] Med.-Chir. Trans., vol. i, p. 216.

[2] Christison on Poisons, p. 539.

Sir George Baker makes an observation of the same nature as that of Dr. Christison. "The custom," says he, "which prevails in many parts of this country of keeping milk in leaden vessels, seems liable to a similar objection, (that of receiving contamination.) One would naturally imagine that it cannot turn sour in such vessels, without dissolving some of the metal. But on applying the *liquor probatorius* to some milk which I had kept in leaden vessels six days, I perceived no such discoloration of it as showed any saturnine solution."[1] I need hardly add, however, that the custom is a dangerous one, and ought to be totally abandoned. It is somewhat curious that more cases of lead poisoning do not arise from this source.

Earthen vessels are generally, more or less, glazed with lead, and acids have been known to corrode the glazing. Dr. Beck, in his work on 'Medical Jurisprudence,' alludes

[1] Med.-Chir. Trans., vol. i, p. 264.

to a case, where a whole family were seized with violent colic, vomiting, and convulsive spasms, by eating some stewed apples which had been kept for some months in a large earthen vessel. The glazing was found corroded, and a solution from the stewed apples gave the usual indications of lead. I have met with a case of a somewhat similar nature in my own practice.

Dr. Hohnbaum mentions an instance of five persons being seized with cohc, and some with palsy, after partaking of a salad, which had been dressed in an earthenware vessel kept for that purpose, and the glazing of which was found destroyed,—an ounce of vinegar remaining in the vessel contained no less than nine grains of the lead. It appears that when the *glaze* is cracked, it is more easily acted upon by acids.[1]

That vinegar may become adulterated with lead in this way, there can be little

[1] Christison, p. 541.

question; but I have no doubt that, in many cases, the vinegar sold in the shops is already impregnated with the metal. On one occasion, being desirous of examining a sediment, which I conceived might contain lead, I poured some acetic acid upon it in order to dissolve it, and then tested it with the sulphuretted hydrogen gas. This produced a dark brown precipitate, but, thinking it possible that the acid itself might contain lead, I afterwards tested the acid in a separate manner, and the same result followed. It is to be regretted that an article which is so commonly employed with our food, should be so easily adulterated.

It appears that the litharge glaze is acted upon by fatty substances as well as by acids; and dripping or fat, baked in a newly-glazed vessel, has been known to occasion attacks of colic. Much depends on the manner in which the glaze is made, as potters may put too much oxide of lead in the composition.

The more common kinds of earthenware, covered with the black glaze, are the most likely to be prejudicial.

Some of the inferior kinds of metallic vessels, which are made of compositions containing lead, are, in all probability, injurions; particularly where vinegar is used for the preparation of food. It is said that a simple mode of discovering the presence of lead, in such cases, is to rub the finger over the surface of the metal, and notice whether it acquires a blackish colour by the contact.

In tinning copper vessels, Sir G. Baker tells us, that the work is not considered finished until covered with a composition in which there is a very large proportion of lead; viz. ten ounces of lead to sixteen of tin. He adds that, in order to discover whether the metal employed for this purpose contains lead, "no other experiment is necessary than to rub the surface of it with a finger;

which, when lead enters the composition, always contracts a livid blackish colour, but is not discoloured when rubbed on pure tin only."[1] In order to determine how far such composition might be objectionable for culinary purposes, he put a mixture, containing butter, salt, water, and vinegar, into a vessel composed of it, and after heating the mixture over the fire, and letting it stand twenty hours in the vessel, it was tested, and found contaminated.

A very curious and interesting case bearing on this subject, is related by Dr. Todd.[2] A man was brought into King's College Hospital in a profound state of coma, which was accompanied by epileptic fits; when he recovered he was found to be palsied in the upper extremities, with a dropping of the wrists; so that when he held out his arms, the hands hung as if lifeless;—the ball of the thumb

[1] Med.-Chir. Trans., vol i, p. 271.

[2] Medical Gazette, 19th December, 1851 (p. 1045).

was wasted, and his grasp was very feeble. The urine was found albuminous, and it was, at first, thought that the complaint was the result of a renal affection. There were circumstances, however, which made Dr. Todd suspect that the complaint depended on the poison of lead. The manner in which the hands dropped at the wrists, reminded him of the painter's palsy; and the gums were found to have the blue line described by Dr. Burton. The blue discoloration was noticed at the margins of the teeth; but where these were imperfect, it was not observed. It was not, however, easy to discover in what way the patient could have been affected with lead, for he was not a house painter,—but a waiter at an inn. Yet the palsy could not have depended on renal disease, for it *preceded* the convulsions, and, it appears, had been attended with colic. It is true that he had been in Devonshire, but he stated that he had never drunk the cyder. It is possible that this man may have taken contaminated water, but Dr. Todd thought it more likely that the complaint had arisen from another cause. "But I think we have a better explanation than this (says he); it appears that a part of his duty has been to clean and keep bright the pewter pots, belonging to the public house to which he is attached: this he does by friction with the hands. Now pewter very commonly contains lead in considerable quantity; and, no doubt, the frequent contact of this with the hands, would lead to a gradual absorption of a sufficient quantity of the metal to produce the poisonous effects; or the repeated frictions might cause the separation of minute metallic particles which might be inhaled." How far this explanation is satisfactory, I will scarcely undertake to determine.

Tanquerel Desplanches mentions the case of a Dr. Corsin, of La Villette, near Paris, who, having been for two nights in a chamber newly painted with white lead, was attacked with all the symptoms of colic; afterwards his head became affected,—then delirium and coma came on, which were eventually fatal.[1] Dr. Percival says,—"A lady of delicate constitution always finds herself affected with the colic, if she sits half an hour in a room which has been lately painted; and a gentleman and his wife, by sleeping in such a chamber, a few years ago, were both violently disordered."[2] I have myself, lately, seen some cases of minor ailments, which I believe were produced by lead, in recently-painted houses. The turpentine, used as a menstruum for oil paints, serves to convey small particles of carbonate of lead to the respiratory organs.

Dr. Christison states that Dr. Taufflieb, of Barr, observed lead colic to arise from the continued use of diachylon plaster, during

[1] British and Foreign Med. Rev., 1840, vol. x, p. 431.
[2] On the Poison of Lead.

eleven weeks, for dressing an extensive ulcer; he goes on to say,—"Such accidents are exceedingly rare, and some auxiliary cause must have favoured the operation of the poison."[1] One case came, however, under my own notice, which seemed to arise from this cause. A little boy had an extensive burn under the arm, which was regularly dressed with adhesive plaster; after a time his body became swelled,—he lost the use of his legs, and suffered from griping pains in the bowels. I at once suspected that he was suffering from the poison of lead, but was unable to trace through what means.

Mr. Mann, of Manchester, who had formerly attended the family, and who was consulted at my request, entered into my views, and suggested that the plaster might be the occasion of the symptoms. It was accordingly given up, and the boy speedily

[1] On Poisons, p. 562.

recovered. I should not omit to state that the granulations of the sore assumed a dark and somewhat sloughy appearance, which I at first attributed to cold,—the weather being very severe at the time,—but I now think that the lead had probably a local influence.

In October, 1851, a servant-lad cut his wrist in cleaning some glass; the wound was extensive, and the skin torn up for some distance. I strapped it over with adhesive plaster, and continued to do so for many days, when the granulations became dark, and as if inclined to slough;—remembering the former case, I substituted some calamine cerate, and a speedy improvement took place.

Whether the mere contact of lead can, under certain circumstances, give rise to the effects which have been described, I am unable to say from my own experience; but some cases are on record, in which, either in this or some other way, the influence of the metal was felt from its external employment.

Dr. Franklin long ago observed that the handling of warm printing types occasioned paralysis of the hands, but he was not quite certain how much of this effect might be due to want of cleanliness on the part of the workmen, by which particles of lead might be swallowed with the food.

Dr. Percival believed that the external application of lead was in itself sufficient.

"Dr. Wall (says Dr. Percival), to whose friendship I am under many obligations, has lately favoured me with the following case:—'I was some years ago called to the son of a plumber in this town (Worcester), a child about two years of age, who had been remarkably healthy till this illness. He had been taken, a few days before I saw him, with violent pains in the bowels, attended with a fever, and convulsive motions in his limbs. These complaints had been attributed to worms, and several medicines had been given unsuccessfully. When I visited him first, I found him paralytic on one side, and delirious. Upon inquiring into the cause of his disorder, and particularly whether the child had been used to go into the room where they melted the lead, I was informed that he did frequently, and that it was a custom with his maid to let him run barefooted along the sheets of lead whilst they were warm, with which he appeared to be much delighted. I did not then hesitate to attribute his present disorder to this cause.'"[1]

The same writer (Dr. Percival) says:—"I have been informed, from undoubted authority, that Dr. A— had a slight paralytic affection of his legs, by the practice of setting his feet every evening on a piece of lead placed near the fire; and that a

[1] On the Poison of Lead, p. 127.

dog, by lying on it, was entirely deprived of the use of his limbs."[1]

It seems to me probable that something may be attributable to particles of lead being swallowed, as Dr. Franklin suggested; but yet I am disposed to think that the frequent contact of lead may itself be injurious.

The accidental mixture of lead with food may sometimes take place, and it may be well to bear in mind the possibility of this occurrence, though it is happily a rare mischance. A remarkable instance is on record, as having occurred in the practice of a Mr. Deering, in London, in October, 1808. Mr. Deering was requested to visit the wife of a respectable tradesman in Aldersgate Street. She had vomited a quantity of bilious matter, and had pain at the stomach,—yet the tongue was clean, the pulse calm, and there was no fever present. Some aperient medicine was given, and an opiate administered after its

[1] On the Poison of Lead, p. 17.

operation, and by these means relief was procured; but the following morning the sickness and pain returned.

A physician was now consulted, who regarded the complaint as "of a rheumatic and spasmodic nature." In a week after this period, a youth, of 16 years of age, became ill with analogous symptoms; but, being removed into the country, got well. A child of 6 years old was next attacked, and the mother, who had in some measure recovered, again fell ill. Three other persons in the family afterwards began to suffer, and suspicion was naturally entertained that the indisposition arose from some poisonous article of food; but minute investigation led to no elucidation of the cause. The lady continued to suffer, but the child was deemed convalescent, and the physician had ceased his visits, when it was seized with convulsions and died. The lady had an infant at the breast, which, being

15 months old, she was advised to wean. This she reluctantly consented to do; but, ten days afterwards, it became costive, and being affected with vomiting and convulsions, suddenly expired. She now became worse herself, and was persuaded to consult an empiric; but as she received no benefit, on the 3d of January, 1809, she took the advice of Mr. Chevalier, an experienced surgeon. He considered her complaint to be chronic rheumatism. He advised the use of clysters, mucilaginous medicines, fomentations, and vesications. These seemed to give more relief than former remedies, and Mr. Chevalier proposed to pay his final visit on the 21st, as she had become so much better as to be able to go about her domestic concerns, and amuse herself with needlework. On the morning of the day mentioned, she rose at ten o'clock, and about an hour afterwards, while standing near the drawers, she suddenly exclaimed,—

"I am dying!"—she was seized with convulsions, which continued until five in the afternoon, when she expired. On the subsequent day Mr. Chevalier, who was an experienced anatomist, examined the body, but could find no trace of disease. With respect to the other three persons named as similarly affected, two, who were removed from the house, recovered; but the third, who was mother-in-law to the lady, died after a lingering illness. The circumstances being mentioned at the Medical and Chirurgical Society, Dr. Adams, Dr. Hamilton, and Mr. Lawrence visited the house, and examined accurately all the culinary articles, but without discovering the source of the unfortunate calamity. At length Dr. Laird, another member of the Medical and Chirurgical Society, who subsequently visited the house, noticed a white powder adhering to a cask which had contained sugar, and which, on examination with the blowpipe, was discovered to be white lead. The cask of sugar had been bought at a sale, and it appears that the cask in which the sugar was put, had formerly contained white lead. Suspicion had not sooner been attached to this article, because a part of it, which had been sent into the country, occasioned no mischief. The immunity, no doubt, arose from the fact, that the portion of the sugar sent away, was derived from the *middle* of the cask, whilst that at the *sides*, to which the lead clung, was reserved for household use.

Besides the *accidental* admixture of lead with sugar, they are sometimes combined in the manufactory, and some objectionable means of purifying sugar with lead were only lately proposed; but I trust they have been abandoned.

It is very probable that many disorders arise from lead contained in fermented liquors. I have frequently noticed that lead pumps are used in public houses, and the first draught of the fluids they contain, must often be extremely prejudicial.—But, in some cases, the water used in brewing is itself objectionable. I once attended a lady who was troubled with a pain in the stomach, which did not yield, nor receive mitigation from the remedies which are accustomed to be found useful. As this lady hàd been previously informed of the injurious influence of lead on water, and had herself taken much interest in the subject, I did not think it necessary to insist on this point. The complaint, however, assumed much resemblance to the affections produced by lead, so that I ventured to suggest the possibility of her illness having this source. But the spring water which supplied the house was remarkably pure, and it was not until some time had elapsed, that it occurred to me that the ale which she drank, and which was brewed at home, might be made from contaminated water. On inquiry, it appeared that this was actually the case. The ale was made from the soft water contained in a lead cistern, and the water was strongly impregnated with lead. After this was pointed out, the lady took no more of the ale, and lost a very troublesome and pertinacious complaint.

I conceive that many persons, who brew their own beer, are in the habit of using soft water in the same manner. The subject appears to me of considerable importance; but there is a practical difficulty in the way of arriving at the chemical evidence, owing to the colour of malt liquor, which interferes with the ready application of the test. Spirits sometimes contain lead derived from the worm of the still. This has been particularly noticed in rum; and there is a paper in the 'Transactions of the London College of Physicians,' by Dr. John Hunter, on the colic which prevailed, from this cause, amongst the soldiers at Jamaica, in 1781-2. Dr. Franklin likewise noticed the contamination of rum at Boston, from the use of lead.

I may notice, summarily, that cheese has been coloured with red lead, and there are cases related where death has been produced by it. A dog was once killed in a very speedy manner by a piece of such poisonous cheese; he had eaten of the rind, and died in convulsions.[1]

The employment of lead counters by the wine dealers has been a fruitful source of mischief. In France, government has more than once forbidden their use by royal *ordonnances.* It is easy to see that the wine spilt on such counters, and afterwards collected in leaden gutters, would be highly deleterious; and yet such wine has been frequently sold. In England, similar counters are not uncommon. The metallic vessels used for measuring liquids are commonly

[1] *Vide* Beck's Medical Jurisprudence, p. 819.

made of compositions into which lead largely enters, and it is possible that, in some few cases, bad effects may arise from them. Whenever lead is employed for the construction of articles designed to contain food or drink, suspicion ought, at least, to be alive, and caution is always necessary.

It is of importance that the toys placed in the hands of children should not be painted; for it is well known that they are in the habit of putting in their mouths whatever amuses them. For the same reason, children ought not to be trusted with the glazed cards, called *Cartes d'Allemagne.*—By the bye, the manufacture of these cards is extremely prejudicial to the workmen. To apply the coating to the paste-board, it is necessary that the workmen remain in an atmosphere loaded with particles of lead. It would be almost desirable that this refinement should be dispensed with.

I have seen Indian-rubber rings, coated

with a whitish polished surface, designed for infants to suck at the period of teething. I put one of these rings, which a lady of my acquaintance had bought for her infant, into a vessel of water, with a few drops of dilute nitric acid, and afterwards tested the water with the sulphuretted hydrogen gas; it gave indications of the presence of lead.[1] I submitted a red ring to the same ordeal, but it was not affected.

A curious case is related by Sir George Baker, which was furnished to him by his friend, Dr. Hanley, and may be interesting in this place.

A gentleman, who had an issue in the thigh, finding that the pea was not sufficiently depressed, applied a small piece of lead, taken from an Indian tea-chest, over the oil-skin which covered the pea; but the

[1] A respectable chemist, Mr. Jackson, of Princess Street, Manchester, also examined this ring, and corroborated the result by a more careful inquiry.

oil-skin was eventually omitted, and the lead placed in immediate contact with the pea. He afterwards began to experience pain and oppression at the *præcordia* and *diaphragm*, which increased to an intolerable degree, when it occurred to him that the lead might be the cause of his suffering, and, upon abandoning its use, speedily lost his complaint. I put a piece of lead, obtained from a similar source, into some rain water, and, after a comparatively short interval, examined the water, and found it to be contaminated.

I have already alluded to the effect of lead on animals. "An intelligent plumber in Manchester," says Dr. Percival, "assures me that he is unable to keep a cat in his house above a month or two. The animal soon sickens, becomes rough in its coat, listless, emaciated, and dies in a short time of *marasmus*. These symptoms he ascribes to the particles of lead scattered upon the floor of his workshop, which, adhering to the feet of the cat, and being licked off, are swallowed, and exert their virulent powers immediately on the stomach and bowels." A gentleman, recently deceased, whose father was a painter, says that he remembers observing, when a child, that the cats in the neighbourhood of the house became frantic from licking the rain water which settled on the casks of lead; he described their screams in the night as perfectly horrible.

To enlarge further on these points would be to deviate from my original design. Sufficient has, perhaps, been said to awaken caution, or to excite interest,—and this is all that I can hope to attain. To enumerate every possible source of contamination would be tedious, if it were possible.—It will be, at any rate, remembered that water, either spring or soft, may be rendered poisonous by lead pumps, by lead cisterns, or by lead pipes.

When a medical man is directly appealed to, as to the propriety of drinking water which has stood in contact with lead, it is true that he is ready to caution the inquirer against so doing; but I know, that in the practice of his profession, he may omit to ask the patient whether he is in the habit of taking such water, or not be sufficiently alive to the possibility of anomalous and obscure complaints arising from this source. It is not enough that the practitioner discover, by accident, the nature of the disease, after a chronic illness, or, perchance, the death of his patient.

C. and J. Adlard, Printers, Bartholomew Close.

By the same Author,

Price 3*s.* 6*d.*

THE

MEDICAL ASPECTS OF DEATH,

AND

THE MEDICAL ASPECTS

OF

THE HUMAN MIND.

LONGMAN & CO., LONDON.

OPINIONS OF THE MEDICAL PRESS.

"Mr. HARRISON, the author of the very interesting little work before us, has succeeded in his attempt to add another stone to the pyramid so well commenced by previous inquirers. The first essay on the 'Medical Aspects of Death' is a truly masterly account of all those appearances which simulate death, and of death itself;—and it is written in so philosophical a spirit, that it cannot but tend to fulfil the dictum of Johnson, that 'he had found physicians to be amongst the most intelligent and well-informed of his friends.' From a production like the present it would be most difficult to find a quotation which would convey an idea of its general tendency; but we extract the following as a specimen of the author's mode of treating the subject. . . . . . . The second essay, which is one of *rare merit*, has been reprinted from Dr. Forbes Winslow's 'Psychological Journal.'" — *Lancet*, Jan. 10, 1852.

"'The Medical Aspects of Death' is an excellently-written essay on the signs of death, the changes the body experiences after death, premature interment, the bodily changes which immediately precede death, the mode in which death takes place, the way in which the various suicidal agents act in inducing death, and the signs of dying. Each of these sections is illustrated by well-told anecdotes, and ornamented with most appropriate quotations. The following extract will convey to our readers a good idea of Mr. Harrison's powers and style. . . . .

"The second essay 'On the Human Mind considered in some of its Medical Aspects,' is well written, and will well repay reading. It was originally published in the 'Psychological Journal.'"—*Medical Times and Gazette*, Jan. 24, 1852.

"In the elegant little volume now before us, bearing the above title, Mr. Harrison, of Manchester, already very favorably known as a medical writer, presents an interesting view of two important aspects of mortality. The latter 'On the Medical Aspects of the Mind of Man,' a most able essay, has already appeared in the pages of our excellent contemporary, the 'Psychological Journal,' and we doubt not has there fallen under the observation of the majority of our readers. The former contains first an excellent *resumé* of the signs of death, a subject which has lately been very fully investigated, chiefly by French physiologists, and the important results arrived at by whom we have recently noticed at length; second, a review of the causes of death, or the mode in which life terminates; and, third, a notice of the antecedent symptoms of death, or the bodily changes which immediately precede it. The entire is written in a highly philosophic spirit, containing throughout, not alone judicious observations on the intimate link between life and death, which do honour to the author, but valuable medical hints. We cordially commend the tone and character of these essays, and we earnestly press their perusal on the profession. Indeed they may be read too, with advantage, by the non-professional public."—*Dublin Quarterly Medical Journal*, February, 1852.

"In this little volume, Mr. Harrison presents us with a couple of remarkably readable and pleasantly-written essays on two subjects, neither of which it is easy to treat pleasantly. In his preface the author *naïvely* observes that he has 'never thought it essential that a book should be dry in order to be useful.' We think that he has produced a useful book; we are sure that he has not added to the stock of dry ones.

"In the first essay, the premonitory signs of death, the several modes in which death is occasioned, and the indications of death having really taken place, are discussed with an absence of disagreeable detail, and yet with a fulness of description, that bespeak a skilful and not unpractised hand. We do not know of any other work in which the unprofessional reader could meet with the same information so intelligibly and pleasingly conveyed, nor in which the medical man would find the subject so appositely garnished with anecdotes and classical illustrations. . . .

"The second essay touches pointedly, but gently, upon the slighter deviations from health of mind, such as, not constituting acknowledged insanity, are still indicative of disorder of the mental balance. To do justice to Mr. Harrison's mode of treating the subject, we should have to transcribe his essay. We need scarcely say that we commend this work to our readers. It is such as we may frequently find convenient to place in the hands of our more intelligent patients. The author has managed to combine the *utile* with the *dulce* in a way *which must ensure success.*" —*Provincial Medical and Surgical Journal*, March 3, 1852.

Also, by the same Author,

A TRACT

ON THE

CONTAMINATION OF WATER WITH LEAD.

Price 6*d.*

LONDON: CHURCHILL.

POPULAR MEDICAL ERRORS.

Price 3*s* 6*d.*

LONDON: LONGMAN & CO.

LETTER TO THE EARL OF SHAFTESBURY

ON

THE INJURIOUS EFFECTS OF THE

MANUFACTURE OF LUCIFER MATCHES,

&c. &c.

MANCHESTER: HAYCRAFT.

Spotted something that isn't quite right?

Let us know and we'll fix it for future reprints. And as a thank you for your diligence, we'll send you a free Sothis book of your choice.

publisher@sothis.press

This page intentionally left blank

Except of course for that line above. And this one.
And whilst we have your attention, perhaps you'd
like to follow us on Instagram @sothis.press. Go on.

Made in the USA
Monee, IL
08 November 2026

67973759R00125